THE TORONTO NOTES PRESENTS

PHARMACOLOGY YOU SEE
A HIGH YIELD PHARMACOLOGY REVIEW FOR HEALTH PROFESSIONALS

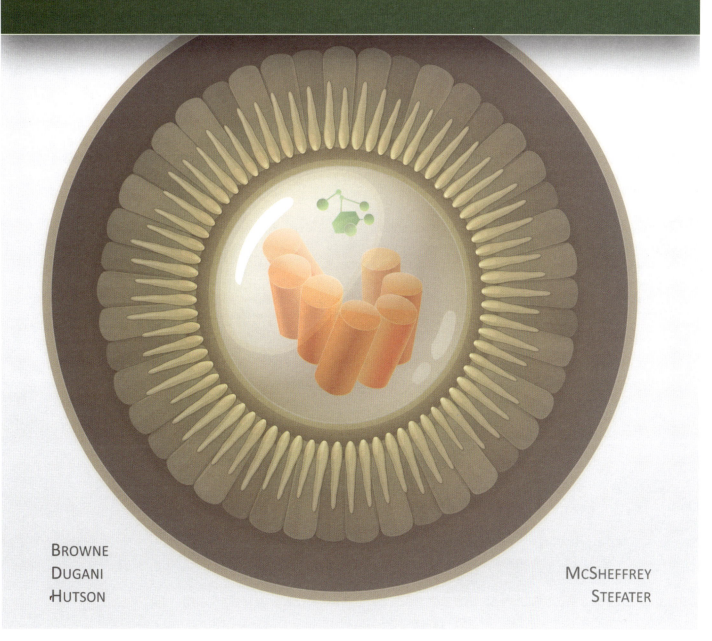

BROWNE
DUGANI
HUTSON

MCSHEFFREY
STEFATER

1st Edition

Copyright © 2011

Typeset and production by Type & Graphics Inc.

All rights reserved. Printed in Toronto, Ontario, Canada.

Pharmacology You See is provided for the sole use of the purchaser. It is made available on the condition that the information contained herein will not be sold or photocopied. No part of this publication may be used or reproduced in any form or by any means without prior written permission from the publisher. Every effort has been made to obtain permission for all copyrighted material contained herein.

Editors-in-chief:	Andrew W. Browne	Gordon G. McSheffrey
	Sagar B. Dugani	Margaret A. Stefater
	Janine R. Hutson	
Cover design:	Walid Aziz, Biomedical Communications program, University of Toronto	
	Representation of the eye looking upon norepinephrine binding to the β-adrenergic receptor	
Figure Illustrations:	Prerna C. Patel, PhD	
Adverse Drug Reaction Icons:	College of Design, Architecture, Art, and Planning, University of Cincinnati	

Notice:
THIS PUBLICATION HAS NOT BEEN AUTHORED, REVIEWED OR OTHERWISE SUPPORTED BY THE MEDICAL COUNCIL OF CANADA NOR DOES IT RECEIVE ENDORSEMENT BY THE MEDICAL COUNCIL AS REVIEW MATERIAL FOR THE MCCQE. THIS PUBLICATION HAS NOT BEEN AUTHORED, REVIEWED OR OTHERWISE SUPPORTED BY THE NATIONAL BOARD OF MEDICAL EXAMINERS U.S.A. NOR DOES IT RECEIVE ENDORSEMENT BY THE NATIONAL BOARD AS REVIEW MATERIAL FOR THE USMLE.

The editors of this edition have taken every effort to ensure that the information contained herein is accurate and conforms to the standards accepted at the time of publication. Due to the constantly changing nature of the medical sciences and the possibility of human error, the reader is encouraged to exercise individual clinical judgement and consult with other sources of information that may become available with continuing research. The authors, editors, and publisher are not responsible for errors or omissions or for any consequences from application of the information in this textbook or associated online resources and make no warranty, expressed or implied, with respect to the currency, completeness, or accuracy of the contents of the publication. In particular, the reader is advised to check the manufacturer's insert of all pharmacologic products before administration.

For more information on *Pharmacology You See*, please visit our website: www.torontonotes.ca

Canadian Cataloguing in Publication Data

ISBN: 978-0-9809397-6-7

Contributors

EDITORS-IN-CHIEF
University of Cincinnati	**Physician Scientist Training Program** Andrew W. Browne, MD, PhD Margaret A. Stefater, PhD	University of Toronto	**MD/PhD Program** Sagar B. Dugani, MSc, PhD Janine R. Hutson, MSc Gordon G. McSheffrey, HBSc

ASSOCIATE EDITOR

University of Toronto — Brian G. Ballios, BSc Eng

CHAPTER AUTHORS

Pharmacology Basics
- University of Cincinnati: Adam Burr, BSc
- University of Toronto: Janine R. Hutson, MSc

Antimicrobial Drugs
- University of Cincinnati: Andrew W. Browne, MD, PhD; Nicholas D. Boespflug, BSc; Adnan Mir, MD, PhD
- University of Toronto: Carolyn C. Tam, BSc, MSc; Jeremy N. Matlow, BMSc

Autonomic Drugs
- University of Cincinnati: Andrew W. Browne, MD, PhD; Amina I. Malik, MD; Margaret A. Stefater, PhD
- University of Toronto: Sanjog Kalra, MD, MSc

Cancer Chemotherapeutics
- University of Cincinnati: Andrew W. Browne, MD, PhD
- University of Toronto: Irene Zelner, BMSc

Cardiovascular Drugs
- University of Cincinnati: Andrew W. Browne, MD, PhD; James A. Stefater, BSc; Margaret A. Stefater, PhD
- University of Toronto: Brian G. Ballios, BSc Eng; Janine R. Hutson, MSc

Central Nervous System Drugs
- University of Cincinnati: Nicole C. Badie, MD; Nicholas D. Boespflug, BSc; Robert B. Hufnagel, MD, PhD; Margaret A. Stefater, PhD; Inuk Zandvakili, BSc
- University of Toronto: Amanda Carnevale, BSc; Monique Moller, MSc; Moumita Sarkar, MSc, PhD; Julianna L. Sienna, HBSc; Seth J. Stern, BMSc

Endocrine Drugs
- University of Cincinnati: Andrew W. Browne, MD, PhD; Jennifer A. O'Malley, MD, PhD
- University of Toronto: Jennifer Galle, MD, HBSc

Gastrointestinal Drugs
- University of Cincinnati: Andrew W. Browne, MD, PhD; Jeeyeon M. Cha, BSc
- University of Toronto: Janine R. Hutson, MSc

Hematological Drugs
- University of Cincinnati: Andrew W. Browne, MD, PhD
- University of Toronto: Brian G. Ballios, BSc Eng

Immune Response Modifiers
- University of Cincinnati: Nicholas D. Boespflug, BSc; Andrew W. Browne, MD, PhD; Norris I. Hollie II, BSc BA
- University of Toronto: Violette M.G.J. Gijsen, MSc

Renal and Urological Drugs
- University of Cincinnati: Andrew W. Browne, MD, PhD; Goutham Vemana, MD; Paul Wiseman, MD
- University of Toronto: Patrina Gunness, HBSc, MSc

Respiratory Drugs
- University of Cincinnati: Andrew W. Browne, MD, PhD; David Simpson, PhD
- University of Toronto: Moumita Sarkar, MSc, PhD

Contributors

Figure Illustrator

Adverse Drug Reaction Icons
University of Cincinnati
- Matt Anthony
- Meagan Brooks
- Maren Carpenter Fearing
- Yongliang Cheng
- Shiyuan Fu
- Nicholas Germann
- Yuan Gu
- Bing Han
- Chris Hendrixson
- Vivek Kalyan
- Jonathan Lowry
- Marnie Meylor
- Chrystal Roggenkamp
- Ryan Rosensweig
- Gaoyan Shi
- Katherine Tans
- Mandy Woltjer
- Zhaoyi Yin

University of Toronto
- Prerna C. Patel, PhD

Special Acknowledgement
University of Cincinnati
- Eleanor Glass, MD
- Robert B. Hufnagel, MD, PhD
- Jeeyeon M. Cha, BSc
- Irfan Asif, MD

University of Toronto
- Julianna L. Sienna, HBSc

FACULTY ADVISORS

University of Cincinnati
Denise Gibson, PhD
Assistant Dean, Academic Support
Associate Professor, Clinical Psychiatry
University of Cincinnati College of Medicine

University of Toronto
Cindy Woodland, PhD
Associate Professor, Department of Medicine
Director, Collaborative Program in Biomedical Toxicology
Senior Lecturer, Department of Pharmacology and Toxicology, University of Toronto

FACULTY REVIEWERS

University of Cincinnati
David J. Draper, MD
Assistant Professor, Good Samaritan Hospital
Resident Program Director, Hematology and Medical Oncology
Staff Physician, Good Samaritan Hospital Cancer Center, Cincinnati Hospital Veterans Affairs

Amit Govil, MD, FASN
Medical Director, Pancreas Transplant Program
Program Director, Renal Transplant Fellowship,
Division of Nephrology and Hypertension
University of Cincinnati Medical Center

Nicole M. Schmidt, PharmD
Transplant Pharmacy Resident,
Department of Surgery, Division of Transplantation
University of Cincinnati Medical Center

Paul M. Zender, MFA
Director, Graduate Program in Design
University of Cincinnati

Contributors

FACULTY REVIEWERS

University of Toronto

Susan Belo, MD, PhD, FRCPC
Anesthesiologist, Sunnybrook Health Sciences Centre
Associate Professor, University of Toronto

Andrea K. Boggild, MSc, MD, DTMH, FRCPC
Physician, Tropical Disease Unit
University Health Network – Toronto General Hospital

Eric X. Chen, MD, PhD, FRCPC
Medical Oncologist
Princess Margaret Hospital
Assistant Professor, Department of Medicine
University of Toronto

Paul Dorian, MD, MSc, FRCPC
Director, Division of Cardiology
St. Michael's Hospital
Professor, Department of Pharmacology and Toxicology, University of Toronto

Linda Dresser, PharmD, FCSHP
Pharmacotherapy Specialist – Antimicrobial Stewardship
University Health Network
Assistant Professor, Leslie Dan Faculty of Pharmacy
University of Toronto

I. George Fantus, MD, BSc, FRCPC
Associate Dean Research, Faculty of Medicine
Professor, Departments of Medicine and Physiology
University of Toronto
Department of Medicine, Mount Sinai Hospital

Yaron Finkelstein, MD
Staff Physician, Hospital for Sick Children,
Associate Professor of Pediatrics, Pharmacology and Toxicology, University of Toronto

Andrea Gershon, MD, MSc, FRCPC
Respirologist, Sunnybrook Health Sciences Centre
Assistant Professor, University of Toronto

Samir C. Grover, MD, MEd, FRCPC
Division of Gastroenterology, St. Michael's Hospital
Assistant Professor, Department of Medicine
University of Toronto

University of Toronto

Geert W. 't Jong, MD, PhD
Clinical Fellow in Clinical Pharmacology,
The MotheRisk Program, Division of Clinical Pharmacology & Toxicology
Hospital for Sick Children

Prateek Lala, MD, MSc
Department of Paediatrics
McMaster University

Bernard Le Foll, MD, PhD, CCFP
Head, Alcohol Dependence Clinic, Centre for Addiction and Mental Health
Associate Professor, University of Toronto

J. Peter McPherson, PhD
Associate Professor, Department of Pharmacology and Toxicology, University of Toronto

John W. Semple, PhD
Professor of Pharmacology, Medicine, Laboratory Medicine & Pathobiology, University of Toronto
Senior Staff Scientist, Keenan Research Centre,
Li Ka Shing Knowledge Institute
Toronto Platelet Immunobiology Group,
St. Michael's Hospital
Adjunct Scientist, Canadian Blood Services

Bernard P. Schimmer, PhD
Professor Emeritus, Department of Pharmacology and Toxicology, University of Toronto

Lisa Thurgur, MSc, MD, FRCPC
Emergency Physician, Undergraduate Coordinator,
Division of Emergency Medicine
Sunnybrook Health Sciences Centre
Clinical Pharmacology Co-Coordinator, Undergraduate Medicine, University of Toronto

Albert H.C. Wong, MD, FRCPC, PhD
Associate Professor, Departments of Psychiatry, Pharmacology and Institute of Medical Sciences
University of Toronto
Research Scientist, Neuroscience Division
Staff Psychiatrist, Schizophrenia Division
Centre for Addiction and Mental Health

Table of Contents

Adverse Drug Reaction Icons 7

Pharmacology Basics 9
    Introduction
    Pharmacokinetics
    Pharmacodynamics

Antimicrobial Drugs 15
    Antibacterials
    Antimycobacterials
    Daptomycin and Antibiotic Mnemonics
    Antifungals
    Antihelminthics
    Antimalarials
    Nonmalarial Antiprotozoals

Autonomic Drugs 35
    Autonomic Nervous System Overview
    The Adrenergic System
    The Cholinergic System
    Glaucoma

Cancer Chemotherapeutics 41
    Antineoplastics
    Molecular Targeted Agents
    Cell Cycle Specific Agents – S Phase
    Cell Cycle Specific Agents – M Phase
    Non-Cell Cycle Specific Agents
    Hormonal Agents

Cardiovascular Drugs 53
    Cardiovascular Electrophysiology
    Antiarrhythmics
    Shock
    Vasodilators and Vasoconstrictors
    Nitrovasodilators
    Sympatholytic/Anti-Adrenergic Drugs
    Non-Autonomic Vasodilators
    Heart Failure
    Antihyperlipidemia Drugs

Central Nervous System Drugs 73
    Anti-Epileptic Drugs
    Parkinson's Disease
    Anesthetics
    Analgesics
    Benzodiazepines
    Anti-Obesity Drugs
    Antipsychotics
    Mood Disorders
    Anxiolytics and Sedative-Hypnotics
    Drugs of Abuse

Endocrine Drugs 105
    Thyroid
    Antidiabetic Drugs
    Corticosteroids

Gastrointestinal Drugs 115
    Introduction
    Inflammatory Bowel Disease
    Anti-Diarrheals
    Laxatives
    Anti-Emetics
    Peptic Ulcer Disease and GERD

Hematological Drugs 125
    Hemostasis and Erythropoiesis
    Thrombolytics
    Anticoagulants
    Antiplatelet Drugs

Immune Response Modifiers 131
    Immune Modulators
    Immunosuppressors
    Immunoenhancers
    Dermatologic Drugs
    Gout

Renal and Urological Drugs 141
    Urinary Continence and Incontinence
    Renin-Angiotensin-Aldosterone System
    Diuretics
    Erectile Dysfunction

Respiratory Drugs 153
    Asthma
    Antihistamines

Appendix A – Tricks for Remembering Drug Names 159

Adverse Drug Reactions Icons

Adverse drug reactions (ADRs) are found with most pharmacological agents at therapeutic and supratherapeutic levels.

This book extends its visual presentation by incorporating icons that represent ADRs with each drug monograph. Our intention is to allow students to remember not only where drugs are on a visually organized page, but also which ADR icons are associated with each agent.

The icons are designed to replace text and require little referral back to the index for description of each icon. Ideally, the reader should be able to simply look at the icon, and "just know what it is." In the index that follows each icon is described and labeled. Throughout the text each icon is used to emphasize those ADRs which are most high yield. Other lower yield ADRs are listed as text. Icons are color-coded according to their effect on organ systems.

Color	System	Color	System
	Blood		Cardiovascular System
	Cancer		Central Nervous System
			Endocrine and Reproductive System
			Internal Organs and Gastrointestinal Tract
			Ocular
			Miscellaneous

Blood

Icon	Adverse Drug Reaction	Icon	Adverse Drug Reaction
	Agranulocytosis/granulocytopenia		Hypertriglyceridemia
	Aplastic anemia		Megaloblastic anemia
	Dehydration		Methemoglobinemia
	Electrolyte imbalance		Neutropenia
	Eosinophilia		Thrombocytopenia
	Hemolytic anemia		Thromboembolism
	Hyperglycemia		

Cancer

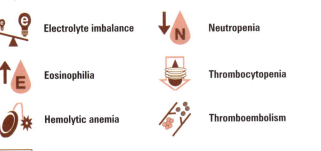

Cardiovascular System

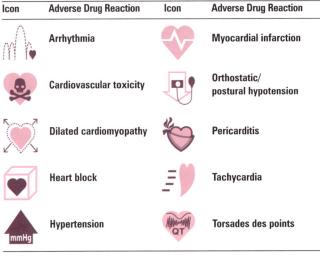

Central Nervous System

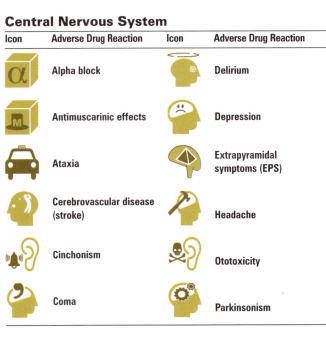

Adverse Drug Reactions Icons

Central Nervous System

Icon	Adverse Drug Reaction	Icon	Adverse Drug Reaction
	Peripheral neuropathy		Stimulation
	Sedation		Suicidal ideation
	Seizure		

Ocular

Icon	Adverse Drug Reaction	Icon	Adverse Drug Reaction
	Blurred vision		Myrdriasis
	Cataracts		Photosensitivity
	Diplopia		Red/green color blind
	Miosis		

Endocrine and Reproductive Systems

Icon	Adverse Drug Reaction	Icon	Adverse Drug Reaction
	Amenorrhea		Irregular bleeding and spotting
	Galactorrhea		Multiple births
	Gynecomastia		Priapism
	Hot flashes		Thyroid problems
	Impotence/decreased libido/sexual dysfunction		

Internal Organs and Gastrointestinal Tract

Icon	Adverse Drug Reaction	Icon	Adverse Drug Reaction
	Constipation		Jaundice
	Diarrhea		Kidney stones
	Gall bladder disease/gallstones		Nausea and vomiting
	Gastric ulcer (Peptic ulcer)		Nephrotoxicity
	GERD (gastroesophageal reflux disease)		Pancreatitis
	GI distress		Pseudo-membranous colitis
	Hemorrhagic cystitis		Pulmonary toxicity
	Hepatoxicity		

Miscellaneous

Icon	Adverse Drug Reaction	Icon	Adverse Drug Reaction
	Bad taste in mouth		Myopathy (muscle ache/weakness)
	Black teeth and bones		Orange body fluids
	Bleeding		P450 (CYP) inducers
	Bone fractures		P450 (CYP) inhibitors
	Contraindicated in pregnancy		Pruritus
	Disuluram (Disulram) reaction		Rash
	Drug induced lupus		Reye's syndrome
	Fever		Skin hyperpigmentation
	Flushing		Stevens-Johnson syndrome
	Gout		Sulfa allergy
	Hirsutism		Tendonitis
	Histamine release		Tyramine
	HIT		Weight gain
	Hypersensitivity		Weight loss
	Malignant hyperthermia		

Pharmacology Basics

Chapter Authors: Adam Burr and Janine R. Hutson

Faculty Reviewer: Cindy Woodland

IN THIS CHAPTER

Introduction 10
    Pharmacology in Medicine
    Terminology
    Drug Dosing
    Bioequivalence
    Absorption Distribution Metabolism Excretion

Pharmacokinetics 11
    Equations
    Absorption
    Distribution
    Elimination
    Metabolism
    Excretion
    1st Order vs. Zero Order Kinetics

Pharmacodynamics 13
    Drug Binding to a Receptor
    Therapeutic Index
    The Dose Response Curve
    Irreversible Antagonist without Spare Receptors
    Irreversible Antagonist with Spare Receptors
    Partial Agonists
    Constant Agonist with Increasing Partial Agonist
    Reversible Competitive Antagonist

Introduction

Pharmacology in Medicine

- Pharmacology in medicine is primarily concerned with:
  - The mechanism(s) of action of a drug
  - The relationship between drug dose and biological effect
  - The site of action of a drug
  - The absorption, distribution, metabolism, and excretion of a drug
  - The relationship between chemical structure and biological activity

Terminology

- **Pharmacokinetics:** deals with the effect of the body on the drug (absorption, distribution, metabolism, and excretion – ADME)

- **Pharmacodynamics:** refers to how drugs act on the body. It often reflects the interaction of a drug with receptors or other drug targets and the effects caused by this interaction

Drug Dosing

The timing of drug dosing can be manipulated to ensure the drug concentration remains above the concentration required for the intended effect of the drug but below the concentration at which adverse drug reactions occur. More frequent, smaller doses will create a tighter range of concentrations than larger doses at longer intervals. Constant infusion of a drug allows one to match the rate of drug administration to the rate of elimination, which will create a nearly constant concentration of drug. It takes approximately 5 half-lives to reach the steady state plasma concentration.

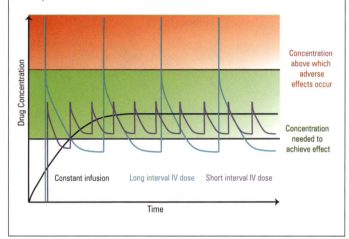

Bioequivalence

For two drugs to be bioequivalent, time to peak concentration, peak concentration, and the area under the curve (AUC) must be approximately the same. Thus, for a generic drug to be bioequivalent to a brand name drug, the above three quantities must be approximately equal. A slow-release version of a drug would not be bioequivalent to the regular preparation because the peak concentration and time to peak would change, by definition.

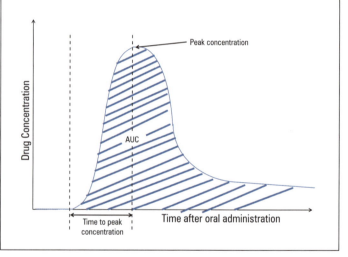

Absorption Distribution Metabolism Excretion

Drugs must cross biological membranes to be absorbed from the GI tract or to reach intracellular targets. A given drug will generally cross a membrane faster than another if it is smaller or more hydrophobic. Charged drugs do not readily cross membranes unless they use a cellular transport protein.

Lungs – Generally, very fast absorption, as in anesthesia or inhaler use.

Liver – The liver generally makes drugs more hydrophillic, so they can be excreted more rapidly. Many drugs are oxidized by the CYP450 system and then conjugated to a very hydrophilic group such as sulfate or glucuronide. Polymorphisms in these enzymes alter metabolism and blood concentration of drugs. The first pass effect occurs when drugs are biotransformed before they reach the systemic circulation. Some drugs are excreted into the bile.

Rectum – Drugs absorbed through the rectum partially bypass the first pass effect but some first pass effect is retained because the upper rectum is part of the portal circulation.

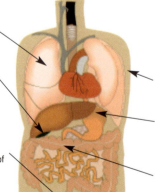

Kidney – Most drugs are eliminated through the urine.

Skin – Slow absorption, but can deliver drugs at very stable levels for a long duration of time.

Stomach – In general, acidic drugs are better absorbed than basic drugs.

Small Intestine – Most drugs are absorbed here because of the rich blood supply and large surface area.

Figure 1. Important Sites of Drug Absorption, Metabolism, and Excretion

Pharmacokinetics

EQUATIONS | EXPLANATIONS

	Equation	Variables	Explanation
Half Life	$k_e = \dfrac{0.693}{t_{1/2}}$	k_e is the elimination rate constant, units of 1/time $t_{1/2}$ is the half life, units of time	This equation can be used to determine the elimination rate constant or the half life when the other parameter is known
Clearance	$Cl = k_e * V_d$	k_e is the elimination rate constant V_d is the volume of distribution	Clearance is the volume of fluid from which a drug is completely removed per unit of time
Volume of Distribution	$V_d = \dfrac{D}{C_o}$	D is the dose of drug C_o is the initial concentration	An apparent volume of distribution larger than the total body water means the drug is distributed to tissue more than blood. A small V_d (~5 L) suggests it is limited to the blood compartment or is bound to plasma proteins
Plasma Drug Concentration	$C = C_0 * e^{-k_e t}$	k_e is the elimination rate constant C_0 is the initial plasma concentration t is the time elapsed	
Bioavailability	$F = \dfrac{AUC_{po}}{AUC_{iv}}$	AUC_{po} is the area under the curve for an oral dose AUC_{iv} is the area under the curve for an intravenous dose	The percentage of drug that enters the systemic circulation in an unchanged form after administration of the product
Therapeutic Index	$TI = \dfrac{LD_{50}}{ED_{50}}$	LD_{50} is the lethal dose in 50% of the population ED_{50} is the effective dose in 50% of the population	This equation yields a unitless ratio of a useful dose and a deadly dose. The higher the TI the safer the drug
Margin of Safety	$MOS = \dfrac{LD_1}{ED_{99}}$	LD_1 the dose which kills 1% of the population ED_{99} is the dose which is effective in 99% of the population	Gives a measure of the relative safety of a drug. Chemotherapy drugs have a low MOS. Safer drugs have higher MOS values
Steady State Concentration (constant infusion)	$C_{ss} = \dfrac{Q}{Cl}$	C_{ss} is the steady state concentration desired Cl is the clearance of the drug Q is the rate of infusion	This equation gives you the infusion rate of drug needed to maintain a given plasma concentration of drug
Steady State Concentration (repeated dosing)	$C_{ss} = \dfrac{F * Dose}{Cl * \tau}$	F is the bioavailability τ is the time between doses	

Remember: When in doubt, the units must work out!

Absorption

- Generally refers to the process by which a drug gets into the bloodstream
- Most drugs are taken by mouth but other common routes include: inhalational, topical, transdermal, intramuscular, intravenous, buccal, intrathecal, and epidural
- Choosing a route depends on many factors and can include availability of formulations, speed of therapeutic onset, location of target organ, drug solubility or absorption

Distribution

- The apparent volume of distribution (V_d) is not a real volume but is a calculation that can be very useful to our understanding of how the drug moves around in the body
  - If the V_d is small, it suggests the drug is confined to the bloodstream
  - If the V_d is large, it suggests the drug can distribute in total body water and perhaps be stored in other tissues, such as fat or muscle
- Most drugs are weak acids or bases, which means that they exist in a charged or uncharged state and this depends on pH
- Uncharged drugs can distribute freely across membranes while charged drugs cannot readily cross membranes without transporters. Charged drugs can thus be trapped in compartments *(ion trapping)*

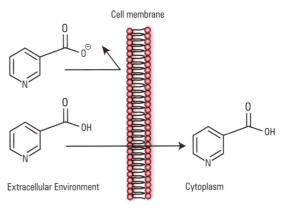

Figure 2. Charged Substances cannot Cross Cell Membranes but Uncharged Substances can do so Freely

Pharmacokinetics

Elimination

- Drug elimination is the combination of both metabolism and excretion
- Clearance is a measure that characterizes the rate of drug removal from the body (total body clearance, TBC) or from a specific organ

Metabolism

- The terms drug metabolism and drug biotransformation can be used interchangeably
- Generally occurs mostly in the liver, but can occur in other tissues such as the kidney and intestine
- The **first pass effect** refers to the biotransformation of a drug before it gets into the systemic circulation and these drugs have less than 100% bioavailability
- Products of drug metabolism may be inactive, active or toxic metabolites
    - For drugs that require biotransformation to become active, the parent compound is called a **prodrug**
- Drug metabolism is generally classified as phase one or two metabolism
    - Phase one metabolism involves oxidation, reduction, or hydrolysis reactions and can involve the cytochrome P450 (CYP450) enzymes
    - Phase two metabolism involves conjugation or synthesis reactions where endogenous substances are added onto the drug molecule
- Drug metabolism generally leads to the molecule being more water soluble than the parent compound and facilitates elimination from the body

Excretion

- Drug excretion is generally thought to occur through the kidneys, but can also occur through bile, feces, exhaled air, skin and breast milk
- Drug transport proteins, such as P-glycoprotein, may influence the rate of drug elimination

1st Order vs. Zero Order Kinetics

1st Order Elimination
- Most drugs are eliminated this way where a constant proportion of drug is eliminated per unit time
- Half the drug is eliminated each $t_{1/2}$
- At 5 $t_{1/2}$, 97% of the drug has been eliminated
- A rule of thumb is that it takes 5 half lives to eliminate a drug

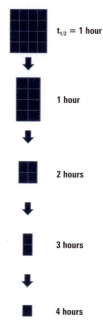

Zero Order Elimination, Saturated Range
- Small doses can produce large effects
- Alcohol behaves this way at typical doses
- Can be slow to leave body because constant amount eliminated per unit time
- Phenytoin and aspirin also have zero order kinetics at higher doses

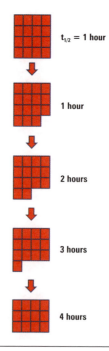

Pharmacodynamics

- Drug targets are often receptors that can be any macromolecule to which a drug selectively binds to initiate its pharmacologic effect
  - Receptors include membrane-bound proteins, intracellular enzymes, ion-linked channels, etc.
  - Most receptors also bind endogenous ligands including hormones and neurotransmitters
  - Drugs can also interact with other macromolecules (such as plasma proteins) where no effect is produced. This is referred to as non-specific binding
- Dose response curves examine the association between drug dose or concentration and the effect of a drug

- Binding of a drug to a particular receptor does not always result in the same effect
  - An **agonist** is a drug that can bind to a receptor and initiate a biological response
  - A **full agonist** can produce a maximal biological response
  - A **partial agonist** has lower efficacy than full agonists and cannot elicit a maximal response even at high drug concentrations
  - An **antagonist** is a drug that can bind to a receptor, but does not cause a response (has zero efficacy)

Drug Binding to a Receptor

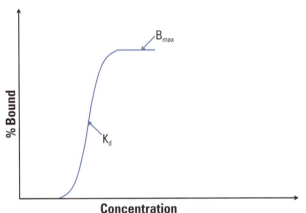

Drug Binding Equation $\quad B = \dfrac{[drug] * B_{max}}{[drug] + K_d}$

Where B_{max} = maximal amount of receptors bound by drug

- Similar to dose response equation
- Binding curve looks similar to dose response curve
- K_d is the drug dissociation constant
- Smaller K_d means tighter binding but does not necessarily mean a greater response
- $K_d = k_{off}/k_{on}$. K_{off} is what differs between most drugs because k_{on} is determined by diffusion

Therapeutic Index

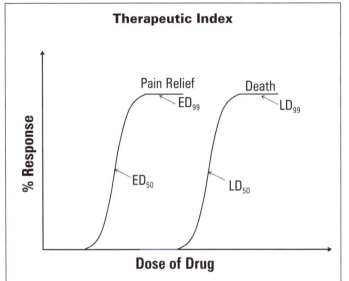

$$TI = \dfrac{LD_{50}}{ED_{50}} \qquad MOS = \dfrac{LD_1}{ED_{99}}$$

- Above curves are used for deriving therapeutic index (TI) and Margin of Safety (MOS)
- TI equation can be remembered as, **TILE TI=L/E**
- TI gives a measure of safety, usually 3-8
- TI <2 requires monitoring
- MOS is essentially a more stringent measurement, 1-3 are common values
- MOS is also referred to as the certain safety factor (CSF)

Pharmacodynamics

The Dose Response Curve

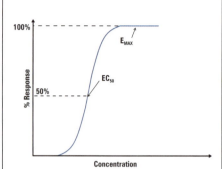

E_{MAX}
- Concentration at which the greatest effect occurs
- E_{MAX} determines therapeutic efficacy
- **NOT related to EC_{50}**

EC_{50}
- EC_{50} is the concentration of drug that gives 50% of maximum response
- EC_{50} is a measure of potency
- Smaller EC_{50} means **more potent** drug
- **NOT related to E_{MAX}**
- EC_{50} does not generally correlate with safety
- If $EC_{50} < K_d$ there are spare receptors

Irreversible Antagonist without Spare Receptors

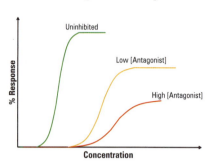

- Irreversible antagonist permanently disables the receptor
- When spare receptors are exhausted, efficacy is lowered
- Overdose cannot be overcome by agonist
- At high doses of irreversible antagonist that leave no spare receptors $K_d = EC_{50}$
- Effect remains after drug is cleared (hours-days), new receptors must be made

Irreversible Antagonist with Spare Receptors

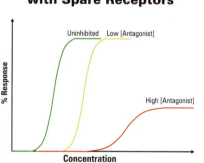

- Spare receptors are receptors in excess of that needed to achieve maximal effect
- Two key effects of spare receptors
  - **Resists desensitization**
  - **Increases sensitivity**
- $K_d > EC_{50}$

Partial Agonists

- Partial agonists can have higher, lower, or equal potency to agonist
- Partial agonists have lower efficacy than full agonists
- Therapeutically advantageous because it allows one to boost the action of the system with room to increase further with full agonist
- Partial agonists can bind either active or inactive receptors

Constant Agonist with Increasing Partial Agonist

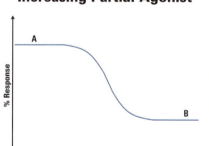

- A partial agonist and full agonist each bind with the same receptor
- In this example a full agonist at constant fixed dose stimulates the receptor to some level of response (A)
- As partial agonist concentration increases, it out-competes the full agonist and displaces the full agonist from the receptor
- Therefore, when sufficient partial agonist is added and displaces all of the full agonist, the maximum response becomes that of the partial agonist (B)

Reversible Competitive Antagonist

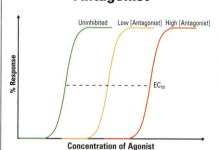

- Competitive, reversible antagonists characterized by **parallel rightward shift of dose** response curve
- **Potency decreases**
- **EC_{50} increases**
- **Efficacy remains constant**
- Can be overcome by sufficiently high concentration of agonist to achieve E_{MAX}

Antimicrobial Drugs

Chapter Authors: Nicholas D. Boespflug, Andrew W. Browne, Jeremy N. Matlow, Adnan Mir and Carolyn C. Tam
Faculty Reviewers: Andrea K. Boggild and Linda Dresser

IN THIS CHAPTER

Antibacterials 17
    Cell Wall Synthesis Inhibitors
    Nucleic Acid Synthesis Inhibitors
    Protein Synthesis Inhibitors

Antimycobacterials 25

Daptomycin and Antibiotic Mnemonics 26

Antifungals 27

Antihelminthics 29

Antimalarials 31

Nonmalarial Antiprotozoals 33

DRUGS IN THIS CHAPTER

Generic Name	US Trade Name	Canadian Trade Name
Albendazole	ALBENZA	
Amikacin	AMIKIN	
Amoxicillin		AMOXIL
Amoxicillin + Carbenicillin	GEOCILLIN	
Amphotericin B		FUNGIZONE
Ampicillin		
Ampicillin + Sulbactam	UNASYN	
Atovaquone + Proguanil		MALARONE
Azithromycin		ZITHROMAX
Aztreonam	AZACTAM, CAYSTON	CAYSTON
Caspofungin		CANCIDAS
Cefazolin	ANCEF, KEFZOL	ANCEF
Cefepime		MAXIPIME
Cefixime		SUPRAX
Cefprozil		CEFZIL
Ceftaroline	TEFLARO	
Ceftazidime		FORTAZ
Ceftriaxone		ROCHEPHIN
Cefuroxime		CEFTIN
Cephalexin		KEFLEX
Chloramphenicol	CHLOROMYCETIN	PENTAMYCETIN
Chloroquine	ARALEN	PLAQUENIL
Ciprofloxacin		CIPRO, CILOXAN
Clarithromycin		BIAXIN
Clindamycin	CLEOCIN	DALACIN C
Clofazimine	LAMPRENE	
Cloxacillin	CLOXAPEN	CLOXI
Dapsone	ACZONE	
Daptomycin		CUBICIN
Dicloxacillin		
Doripenem		DORIBAX
Doxycycline		VIBRAMYCIN
Ertapenem		INVANZ
Erythromycin	ERYC, ERY-TAB	ERYC
Ethambutol	MYAMBUTOL	ETIBI
Fluconazole		DIFLUCAN
Flucytosine	ANCOBON	
Gentamicin		GARAMYCIN
Griseofulvin	FULVICIN	
Imipenem + Cilastatin		PRIMAXIN
Iodoquinol	YODOXIN	DIODOQUIN

DRUGS IN THIS CHAPTER (continued)

Generic Name	US Trade Name	Canadian Trade Name
Isoniazid + Rifampin + Pyrazinamide	RIFATER	
Itraconazole	SPORANOX	
Ivermectin	STROMECTOL	MECTIZAN
Ketoconazole	NIZORAL	
Levofloxacin	LEVAQUIN	
Linezolid	ZYVOX	ZYVOXAM
Mebendazole	VERMOX	
Mefloquine	LARIAM	
Meropenem	MERREM	
Methicillin	STAPHCILLIN	
Metronidazole	FLAGYL	
Minocycline	MINOCIN	
Moxifloxacin	AVELOX, VIGAMOX	
Nafcillin		
Norfloxacin	NOROXIN	
Nystatin	MYCOSTATIN	
Ofloxacin	OCUFLOX	
Oxacillin		
Penicillin	BICILLIN, PERMAPEN	BICILLIN, CRYSTAPEN
Pentamidine	PENTAM, NEBUPENT	
Piperacilin + Tazobactam	ZOSYN	TAZOCIN
Polymyxin B + bacitracin + neomycin	NEOSPORIN	
Polymyxin B + gramicidin	POLYSPORIN	
Polymyxin B + neomycin + dexamethasone	MAXITROL	
Praziquantel	BILTRICIDE	
Primaquine	PRIMAQUINE	
Pyrantel		COMBANTRIN
Pyrazinamide		TEBRAZID
Pyrimethamine	DARAPRIM	
Quinine	QUINAMM	
Rifabutin	MICOBUTIN	
Rifampin	RIFADIN	
Streptomycin		
Sulfadiazine	THERMAZENE, SILVADENE	FLAMAZINE
Sulfamethoxazole + Trimethoprim	BACTRIM	BACTRIM, SEPTRA
Telavancin	VIBATIV	
Terbinafine	LAMISIL	
Tetracycline	SUMYCIN	TETRA
Ticarcillin + Clavulanic Acid	TIMENTIN	
Tigecycline	TYGECIL	
Tobramycin	TOBREX, TOBI	TOBREX
Trimethoprim	PROLOPRIM	
Vancomycin	VANCOCIN	
Voriconazole	VFEND	

Antibacterials – Cell Wall Synthesis Inhibitors

Cell Wall Synthesis
The bacterial cell wall is synthesized through the linkage of peptidoglycan at both the carbohydrate (transglycosylation) and peptide (transpeptidation) moieties by penicillin-binding proteins (PBPs)

β-LACTAMS
- Penicillins
- Cephalosporins
- Carbapenems
- Monobactams

MOA
- Inhibit cell wall synthesis by:
  - Binding to PBPs in the bacterial membrane
  - Inhibiting the cross-linking of peptidoglycan
  - Activating bacterial autolytic enzymes

PK
- Distribute throughout the body EXCEPT many have limited distribution to the eye, prostate and CNS
- Renal elimination (filtration and secretion)
  - EXCEPT **CLOXACILLIN** and **CEFTRIAXONE** (fecal elimination)
  - Tubular secretion is inhibited by **PROBENECID** (increased duration of antibiotic action and risk of toxicity)

ADRs
- Hypersensitivity
  - Immediate: anaphylaxis
  - Accelerated: fever, rash, urticaria, angiodema
  - Late: rash, serum sickness, interstitial nephritis, hemolytic anemia
- Pseudomembrane colitis
- With high doses:
  - Seizures and encephalopathy
  - Cation toxicity (Na^+ and K^+ in salts) especially in the context of renal and cardiovascular disease

Mechanisms of Resistance to β-lactams
- β-lactamases cleave the β-lactam ring
- Mutations in PBPs decrease affinity of drug
- Mutations in bacterial outer membrane porins decrease influx of drug
- Increased efflux of drug by bacterial efflux transporters

β-LACTAMASES VARY IN STRENGTH
- Weakest – plasmid encoded
- Moderate – chromosomally encoded
- Strongest – inducible chromosomally encoded [in species of *Pseudomonas*, *Enterobacter* and *Serratia* (PES)]

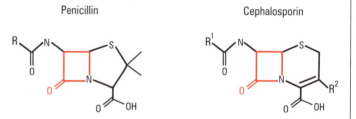

Figure 1. Penicillin and Cephalosporin (β-lactam ring highlighted in red)

> Significant cross-reactivity between penicillins and cephalosporins/carbapenems → if a patient is allergic to one penicillin, assume he or she is allergic to all cephalosporins and carbapenems

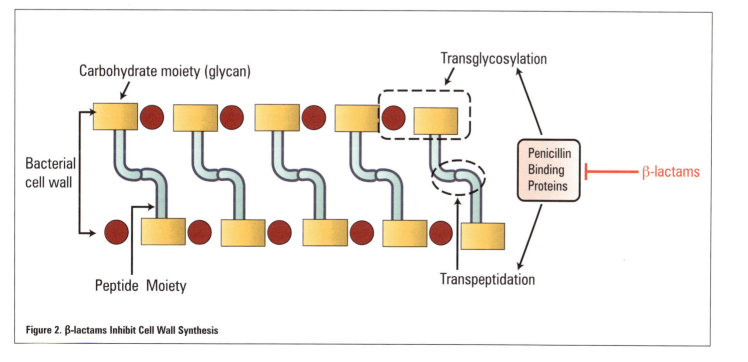

Figure 2. β-lactams Inhibit Cell Wall Synthesis

Antibacterials – Cell Wall Synthesis Inhibitors

Narrow Spectrum Penicillins

PENICILLIN (β-LACTAMASE SENSITIVE)
(a) **PENICILLIN G** (IV administration – you G-IV-e penicillin G via IV)
(b) **PENICILLIN V** (acid stable → PO administration for oropharyngeal infections)

SPECTRUM
- Gram positive cocci and rods
- Gram negative rods
- Spirochetes

USES
- DOC for syphilis (*Treponema pallidum*)
- DOC for strep throat (*Streptococcus pyogenes*)
- Meningococcal disease (*Neisseria meningitidis*)
- Actinomycosis (*Actinomyces* spp.)
- Diptheria (*Corynebacterium diphtheriae*)
- Pneumonia (*Streptococcus pneumoniae*)

RESISTANCE: β-lactamase-sensitive
- β-lactamases produced by:
  - Most Gram negative bacteria
  - Most intracellular bacteria
  - Most staphylococci
- *N. meningitidis*, *Streptococcus pneumoniae* produce altered PBP

CLOXACILLIN, DICLOXACILLIN, METHICILLIN, NAFCILLIN, OXACILLIN
(β-LACTAMASE-RESISTANT PENICILLINS)
USES
- Narrow spectrum – Gram positive cocci only
- *Staphylococcus* spp. (**give "naf" for staph**)

ADRs
- Interstitial nephritis

RESISTANCE
- Methicillin-resistant *Staphylococcus aureus* (MRSA) produce altered PBP with lower affinity for penicillin

NOTES
- Bulky **R** group makes them resistant to the β-lactamase in *Staphylococcus* spp.
- **METHICILLIN** not available for clinical use, but still used in laboratories to identify resistant bacteria
- **OXACILLIN** is now commonly used to identify resistant bacteria [Also known as oxacillin-resistant *Staphylococcus aureus* (ORSA)]

Broad Spectrum Penicillins

TICARCILLIN, PIPERACILLIN
(β-LACTAMASE SENSITIVE)

SPECTRUM
- More activity against Gram negative bacteria than other penicillins
  - PEKS = *Pseudomonas, Enterobacter, Klebsiella, Serratia*
- Less activity against Gram positive bacteria

USES
- Serious infections caused by Gram negative bacteria:
  - Bacteremia
  - Pneumonia (e.g. in cystic fibrosis patients)
  - Infections following burns
  - Urinary tract infections

RESISTANCE: β-lactamase sensitive
- Inducible chromosomal β-lactamases
  - PES (*Pseudomonas, Enterobacter, Serratia*) and Gram negative
- Commonly used with β-lactamase inhibitors
  (e.g. **PIPERACILLIN/TAZOBACTAM**)

NOTES
- Can be used synergistically with aminoglycosides

AMINOPENICILLINS

AMOXICILLIN, AMPICILLIN
SPECTRUM
- Similar to penicillin with increased activity against Gram negative bacteria (SMEESHL)
- "Amoxicillin is SMEESHL" (special)
  - *Salmonella* spp.
  - Meningococci (*N. meningitidis*)
  - Enterococcus
  - *Escherichia coli* (some)
  - *S. pneumoniae*
  - *Haemophilus influenzae* (When used in combination with a β-lactamase inhibitor)
  - *Listeria monocytogenes*

USES
- Acute otitis media, sinusitis, UTI, URTI and salmonellosis
- Human or animal bites
- *H. pylori* (+ macrolide ± proton pump inhibitor)
- Meningitis caused by *L. monocytogenes*

ADRs
- Non-allergic rash

RESISTANCE: β-lactamase-sensitive
- Commonly used with β-lactamase inhibitors
  (e.g. **AMOXICILLIN/CLAVULANATE**)

β-LACTAMASE INHIBITORS
The only penicillins found in formulations with a β-lactamase inhibitor are **AMOXICILLIN, AMPICILLIN (AMINOPENICILLINS) and **TICARCILLIN, CARBENICILLIN** and **PIPERACILLIN**

CLAVULANIC ACID, SULBACTAM, TAZOBACTAM
MOA
- "Suicide" inhibitors – bind irreversibly to catalytic site of β-lactamases

SPECTRUM
- Most effective against plasmid-encoded β-lactamases
- Some activity against chromosomal β-lactamases
- Poor activity against inducible chromosomal β-lactamases of PES

Antibacterials – Cell Wall Synthesis Inhibitors

Cephalosporins
Used against bacteria with high resistance to penicillin (e.g. *Streptococcus pneumoniae, Neisseria gonorrhoeae*)

- Similar to penicillins in β-lactam core, MOA, elimination, and ADRs
- Rules for cephalosporins:
  (1) As generation increases:
    a. More active against Gram negative bacteria
    b. More resistant to β-lactamases
    c. May be less active against Gram positive bacteria
  (2) Oral cephalosporins are less potent and narrower in spectrum
  (3) Only 3rd generation cephalosporins reach therapeutic levels in the CNS
- All cephalosporins are broader spectrum than penicillins → increased risk of superinfection
- None are active against MRSA, *Enterococcus* spp., or *L. monocytogenes*

SPECTRUM/USES
- Can be used as alternative to penicillin for patients with **mild** penicillin hypersensitivity

ADRs
- Hypersensitivity
  - 10% cross-reactivity with penicillin allergy → if a patient has a major allergy to penicillin, do not use a cephalosporin – use a different class
  - Variable presentation: mild rash to anaphylactic shock
  - Less common than penicillin
- Interstitial nephritis, enhances the nephrotoxicity of aminoglycosides

1st Generation

SPECTRUM
- Most Gram positive cocci, except enterococci and MRSA
- More active against Gram positive bacteria than AMOXICILLIN
- Active against a few Gram negative rods (CEFAZOLIN > CEPHALEXIN)

CEFAZOLIN
USES
- Surgical prophylaxis
- Substitute for anti-staphylococcal penicillins (e.g. DICLOXACILLIN/CLOXACILLIN) in mildly allergic patients

CEPHALEXIN
USES
- Mild infections of skin and soft tissue caused by *S. aureus, S. pyogenes*
- Urinary tract infections

2nd Generation

CEFUROXIME, CEFPROZIL
SPECTRUM
- Less activity against Gram positive cocci than 1st generation, more activity against Gram negative bacteria
- Resistant to β-lactamases produced by most Gram positive and Gram negative bacteria
- Susceptible to inducible chromosomal β-lactamases (PES)
- *Haemophilus influenzae*

NOTES
- Largely displaced by 3rd generation cephalosporins

3rd Generation

SPECTRUM
- Less activity against Gram positive than 2nd generation cephalosporins
- Retain activity against *Streptococcus* spp. (Gram positive)
- More activity against Enterobacteriaceae (Gram negative)
- Active against many bacteria with mutated PBP
- Resistant to β-lactamases, except inducible chromosomal β-lactamases (PES)

PK
- Penetrate into CSF

CEFTRIAXONE
USES
- Serious infections by Gram negative bacteria that are resistant to other β-lactams
- DOC for neisserial infections
  1. Meningitis in people over 3 months and non-compromised adults
  2. Gonorrhea
- DOC for
  3. Pneumonia (+ macrolide for intracellular bacteria)

CEFIXIME
USES
- Acute otitis media
- Upper respiratory tract infections
- Bronchitis
- Urinary tract infections

CEFTAZIDIME
USES
- Infections caused by *Pseudomonas* spp. (+ aminoglycoside)
- Has weaker activity against Gram positive compared to other 3rd generation cephalosporins

4th Generation

CEFEPIME, CEFTAROLINE
SPECTRUM
- Among cephalosporins, the most resistant to β-lactamases – even inducible chromosomal β-lactamases
  - Poor inducer of and, therefore, relatively resistant to inducible chromosomal β-lactamases
- Gram positive bacteria (*S. aureus, Streptococcus* spp.)

USES
- Empirical treatment of nosocomial infections where resistance to other antibiotics is anticipated

Antibacterials – Cell Wall Synthesis Inhibitors

Carbapenems

IMIPENEM/CILASTATIN
MEROPENEM, ERTAPENEM, DORIPENEM

MOA
- Binds PBP → inhibits cell wall synthesis

SPECTRUM: Broadest spectrum β-lactam antibiotic
- Active against most Gram positive and Gram negative bacteria, including anaerobes
  - Resistant to most β-lactamases
- Not active against MRSA or most enterococci

USES
- Limited by ADRs (one of the last resort drugs when other drugs have failed)
  - Nosocomial infections with multidrug-resistant bacteria (PES + *Acinetobacter* spp.)
  - Mixed infections
- DOC for *Enterobacter* infections

PK
- **IMIPENEM** is degraded to a toxic metabolite by dihydropeptidase I in the proximal renal tubular brush border
  - Administered with **CILASTATIN**, which inhibits renal dihydropeptidase → decreased renal toxicity, increased $t_{1/2}$
- **MEROPENEM** is resistant to degradation by dihydropeptidase

ADRs
- Gastrointestinal (nausea, vomiting, diarrhea)
- Seizures (**IMIPENEM** > **MEROPENEM**)
- Rash, drug fever (cross-reactive with penicillins)

Monobactams

AZTREONAM

MOA
- Binds to PBP3 → inhibits cell wall synthesis

SPECTRUM
- Active against aerobic Gram negative bacteria, including *Pseudomonas* spp.
- Active against some facultative anaerobes (e.g., *Klebsiella, Serratia*)
- No activity against Gram positive or obligate anaerobes

USES
- No cross reactivity with penicillins → can be used in patients who are severely allergic to penicillins or cephalosporins
- Alternative for patients with renal insufficiency who cannot handle aminoglycosides

PK
- Very short $t_{1/2}$ (1.7 hours)

ADRs
- Gastrointestinal upset
- Transient elevation of liver enzymes

 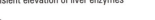

NOTES
- Synergistic with aminoglycosides

Non β-lactam Cell Wall Inhibitors

Polymyxins

POLYMYXIN B

MOA
- Bind to membrane phospholipids and disrupt membrane integrity → leakage of intracellular constituents

SPECTRUM
- Active against Gram negative rods, including *P. aeruginosa*
- Not active against *Proteus, Serratia*, Gram negative cocci

USES
- Serious infections caused by susceptible Gram negative bacteria where other drugs are ineffective or contraindicated
- Ocular infections (topical)

ADRs
- Systemic:
  - Neurotoxicity
    - Dizziness, blurred vision, vertigo
    - Paresthesias
    - Peripheral neuropathy
  - Nephrotoxicity (acute renal tubular necrosis)

Glycopeptides

VANCOMYCIN, TELAVANCIN

MOA
- Binds to D-alanyl-D-alanine terminus of cell wall precursors → inhibits transglycosylation of cell wall mucopeptides
  - Acts at step in cell wall synthesis upstream of penicillins
- Bactericidal for dividing microorganisms

SPECTRUM
- Gram positive bacteria only
- Extracellular bacteria only

USES
- Drug of last resort
- Serious infections caused by multidrug-resistant Gram positive organisms
  - MRSA
  - Pseudomembranous colitis (alternative to **METRONIDAZOLE**)
- Patients with severe allergy to penicillin

PK
- Poor oral absorption
  - IV administration for systemic infection
  - PO administration for GI infection (e.g. *Clostridium difficile*)
- Renal excretion
- Moderate $t_{1/2}$ (6-9 hours)

ADRs
- "Red-man syndrome"
  - Diffuse flushing, erythematous rash of face, neck, and upper torso due to mast cell degranulation and histamine release
  - Prevent by using slow infusion rate, antihistamines
- Ototoxicity (usually irreversible)
  - Increased risk when used in combination with other ototoxic drugs
- Nephrotoxicity (usually reversible)
  - Increased risk when used in combination with other nephrotoxic drugs (e.g. aminoglycosides)
- Thrombophlebitis
- Chills, fever, neutropenia

RESISTANCE
- Altered target → decreased affinity:
  - Amino acid change from D-alanyl-D-alanine to D-alanyl-D-lactate or D-alanyl-D-serine
- Vancomycin-resistant *Enterococcus* (VRE)

Antibacterials – Nucleic Acid Synthesis Inhibitors

METRONIDAZOLE

MOA (Metro – Pro – Nitro)
- **PRODRUG** that is activated by **nitroreductase**
- Highly reactive nitro radicals and metabolites target and damage DNA and inhibit nucleic acid synthesis

SPECTRUM
- Anaerobic bacteria
  - *Bacteroides fragilis*
  - *Clostridia* spp.
    - *C. perfringens* (gas gangrene)
    - *C. botulinum* (botulism)
    - *C. tetani* (tetanus)
    - *C. difficile* (pseudomembranous colitis)
- *Gardnerella vaginalis*

USES
- Acne rosacea (topical)
- DOC for brain abscesses
- Infections below the diaphragm ("use **METRO** below")
- *H. pylori* (**METRONIDAZOLE** + **BISMUTH SUBSALICYLATE** + **AMOXICILLIN/ TETRACYCLINE**)

PK
- Moderate $t_{1/2}$ (8 hours)

ADRs
- Metallic taste
- Nausea
- Dizziness
- Discolored (darkened) urine
- Peripheral neuropathy (rare)
- P450 (CYP2C9) inhibitor

DRUG INTERACTIONS
- Disulfiram-like reaction when consumed with alcohol

NOTES
- See Nonmalarial Antiprotozoal section

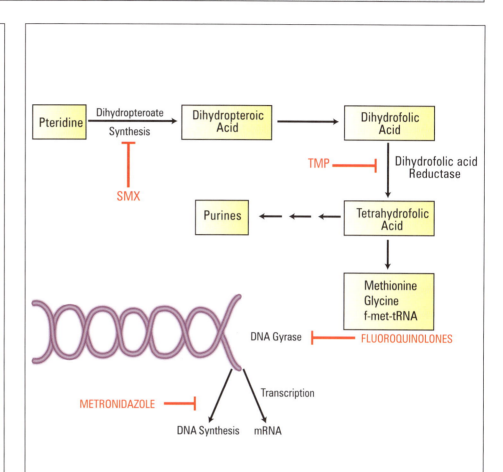

Figure 3. Mechanism of Action of Bacterial Nucleic Acid Synthesis Inhibitors

Antibacterials – Nucleic Acid Synthesis Inhibitors

Fluoroquinolones

CIPROFLOXACIN, NORFLOXACIN, OFLOXACIN, MOXIFLOXACIN, LEVOFLOXACIN

MOA
- Inhibit DNA gyrase (topoisomerase II) and topoisomerase IV → supercoiled DNA → inhibit bacterial synthesis of DNA and RNA

SPECTRUM
- **CIPROFLOXACIN, NORFLOXACIN**
  - Gram negative aerobes
  - Mycobacteria
  - Intracellular organisms (*Legionella, Mycoplasma, Chlamydia, Brucella*)
- Respiratory (**LEVOFLOXACIN, MOXIFLOXACIN, OFLOXACIN**) have expanded coverage to include:
  - Some Gram positive bacteria: staphylococci, streptococci, enterococci

USES
- Urinary tract infections, gastroenteritis caused by susceptible organisms
- Chronic prostatitis
- Chronic osteomyelitis
- Community-acquired pneumonia (respiratory fluoroquinolones only)
- Anthrax prophylaxis and treatment (*Bacillus anthracis*)

ADRs
- Gastrointestinal upset
- Headache, dizziness
- Tendonitis, tendon rupture
- Rash, photosensitivity

DRUG INTERACTIONS
- Absorption decreased by di- and trivalent ions (e.g. Ca^{2+}, Mg^{2+}, iron)
- P450 inhibitor (CYP1A2 and 3A4)

RESISTANCE
- Altered topoisomerase binding site
- Reduced bacterial permeability
- Efflux mechanisms

Sulfonamides

SULFAMETHOXAZOLE (SMX)
SULFADIAZINE

MOA
- Structural analogs of para-aminobenzoic acid (PABA)
  - Bacteria require PABA to synthesize folic acid
- Competitively inhibit dihydropteroate synthase → interfere with bacterial utilization of PABA → inhibit folate synthesis
  - Folate is required for DNA, RNA, and protein synthesis

SPECTRUM: Broad
- Active against Gram positive bacteria, including staphylococci, streptococci, and *L. monocytogenes*, but not enterococci
- Active against Gram negative bacteria
- *Nocardia*
- *Chlamydia*

USES
- Often combined with **TRIMETHOPRIM** (see **TMP/SMX**)
- Silver **SULFADIAZINE** cream – adjunct to prevent sepsis in burn patients (**SULFADIAZINE** is only used topically)

PK
- Moderate $t_{1/2}$ (5-11 hours)

ADRs
- **Hypersensitivity** (highest incidence among all antibiotics)
  - Dermatological: rash, pruritus, photosensitivity, Stevens-Johnson syndrome, toxic epidermal necrolysis
  - Interstitial nephritis → eosinophilia
  - Hepatotoxicity (increased risk in patient with G6PD deficiency)
- Hemolytic anemia (especially in patients with G6PD deficiency)
- Bone marrow suppression
- **Kernicterus in neonates** (when given to mother near term or when given directly to neonate)
  - **SMX** displaces bilirubin from binding sites on serum albumin → unconjugated bilirubin is free to pass into CNS (immature BBB)
  - Bilirubin deposited in cell bodies, especially in the basal ganglia → neurotoxicity
- P450 inhibitor (CYP2C9)

TRIMETHOPRIM (TMP)

MOA
- Structural analog of pteridine ring of dihydrofolate
- Inhibits dihydrofolate reductase (DHFR) → inhibits production of tetrahydrofolate
  - Tetrahydrofolate is an essential cofactor in one-carbon transfer reactions, which are involved in amino acid and nucleic acid metabolism

SPECTRUM
- Similar to sulfonamides + enterococci

PK
- Moderate $t_{1/2}$ (10 hours)

ADRs
- Megaloblastic anemia (due to inhibition of folate metabolism)
  - Treat with supplemental folic acid
- Leukopenia, granulocytopenia
- Maculopapular rash
- Increased serum creatinine (**TMP** inhibits tubular secretion of creatinine)
- P450 inhibitor (CYP2C9)

TMP/SMX
- Synergistic inhibition of folate metabolism

USES
- DOC for:
  - Upper and lower respiratory tract infections:
    - Acute otitis media
    - Sinusitis (adults)
    - Chronic bronchitis
  - Pneumocystis pneumonia
  - Prostatitis
  - Recurrent urinary tract infections
- Alternative drug for:
  - Typhoid fever (*Salmonella typhi*)
  - Shigellosis (*Shigella* spp.)
  - Traveler's diarrhea

RESISTANCE
- Altered dihydropteroate synthase with lower affinity for sulfonamides
- Decreased permeability or active efflux
- Increased production of endogenous substrate (i.e., PABA)

Antibacterials – Protein Synthesis Inhibitors

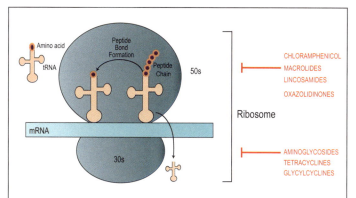

Figure 4. Mechanism of Action of Protein Synthesis Inhibitors

Aminoglycosides

GENTAMICIN, NEOMYCIN, AMIKACIN, TOBRAMYCIN, STREPTOMYCIN

MOA
1. Diffuses across outer membrane of Gram negative bacteria
   a. Synergy with β-lactams (weaken cell wall for better entry)
2. Transport across inner membrane requires O_2 (aerobes only)
3. Binds irreversibly to 30S subunit of bacterial ribosome →
   a. Interferes with formation of initiation complex
   b. Causes misreading of mRNA
   c. Stops translocation

SPECTRUM
- Aerobes only
- Mainly extracellular Gram negative rods
- Some Gram positive (when combined with a cell wall-active agent)

USES
- Severe infections caused by Gram negative rods
- Urinary tract infections caused by *E. coli*
- Bacterial endocarditis caused by susceptible organisms (+ cell wall-active agent)

PK
- Renal excretion
- Short $t_{1/2}$ (1.5 to 2 hours)

ADRs (narrow therapeutic index, therapeutic drug monitoring)
- Nephrotoxicity (accumulation in proximal tubular cells ↑ cell damage)
  - Acute tubular necrosis is rare
  - Usually reversible
- Ototoxicity (may be potentiated by concurrent use of loop diuretics)
  - Vestibular: **STREPTOMYCIN, GENTAMICIN, TOBRAMYCIN**
  - Cochlear, auditory: **AMIKACIN, NEOMYCIN, TOBRAMYCIN**
  - Irreversible, unless detected early
- Neuromuscular blockade (at high dose, still rare)
  - Inhibit presynaptic release of acetylcholine
  - Reduce postsynaptic sensitivity

RESISTANCE
- Mainly due to inactivation by aminoglycoside-modifying enzymes
- Mutation in 30S subunit
- Natural resistance due to failure of drug to penetrate the inner membrane

Macrolides

MOA
- Bind reversibly to 50S subunit of bacterial ribosome → inhibit translocation of peptidyl-tRNA

SPECTRUM
- Mainly Gram positive cocci and rods
- Generally inactive against Gram negative, except *Bordetella pertussis*, *Campylobacter*, *Helicobacter*, and *Neisseria*
- Atypical organisms: *Chlamydophila*, *Legionella*, *Mycoplasma*

USES
- Streptococcal infections in patients allergic to penicillin
- DOC for atypical/walking pneumonias caused by:
  - *Mycoplasma*
  - *Legionella*
  - *Chlamydophila pneumoniae*
  - *Corynebacterium*
- DOC for prophylaxis and treatment of disseminated *Mycobacterium avium complex* and *M. avium intracellulare* (+ other drugs)
- Pertussis (*B. pertussis*)

RESISTANCE
- Efflux transporter
- Ribosomal protection by constitutive or inducible methylases
- Drug inactivation by esterases
- Mutation of 50S subunit

CLARITHROMYCIN
USES (DOC)
- *H. pylori* (+ **AMOXICILLIN** + proton pump inhibitor)
- Prophylaxis and treatment of disseminated *M. avium complex* and *M. avium intracellulare* (+ other drugs)

PK
- Moderate $t_{1/2}$ (3-9 hours)

ADRs
- Gastrointestinal (nausea, vomiting, dyspepsia, abdominal pain, diarrhea)
- Abnormal taste
- Headache
- P450 inhibitor (CYP3A4)

AZITHROMYCIN
- DOC for chlamydia
- *Mycoplasma* infections
- *Moraxella catarrhalis*
- Acute pelvic inflammatory disease caused by *Neisseria gonorrhoeae*
- Prophylaxis and treatment of disseminated *M. avium complex* and *M. avium intracellulare* (+ other drugs)

PK
- Very long $t_{1/2}$ (40 to 68 hours)

ERYTHROMYCIN
USES (DOC)
- *B. pertussis*
- Chlamydia in pregnant women

PK
- Short $t_{1/2}$ (1 to 1.5 hours)

ADRs
- GI distress (most common cause of non-compliance)
- Cholestatic hepatitis (jaundice may be accompanied by fever, leukocytosis, eosinophilia, elevated liver enzymes)
- Cardiac arrhythmia (QT prolongation with ventricular tachycardia)
- Reversible ototoxicity (tinnitus, deafness)
- P450 inhibitor (CYP3A4)

Antibacterials – Protein Synthesis Inhibitors

Lincosamides

CLINDAMYCIN

MOA
- Binds reversibly to 50S ribosomal subunit → prevents translocation of peptidyl tRNA from acceptor site to donor site

SPECTRUM
- Most aerobic Gram positive cocci
- Active against **anaerobes**
  - *B. fragilis*
  - *Fusobacterium*
  - *C. perfringens*
- Not active against most aerobic Gram negative bacteria

USES: Infections above the diaphragm
- Alternative to β-lactams/macrolides for prophylaxis of infective endocarditis
- Acne vulgaris (topical)
- Anaerobic infections

PK
- Short $t_{1/2}$ (1.5-5 hours)

ADRs
- Gastrointestinal distress (diarrhea, nausea, vomiting, abdominal pain)
- Pseudomembranous colitis
- Skin rash
- Fever

Oxazolidinones

LINEZOLID

MOA
- Binds reversibly to 50S ribosomal subunit → prevents formation of 70S initiation complex

SPECTRUM
- Mainly Gram positive cocci and rods, including multidrug-resistant streptococci, staphylococci, and enterococci
- Not active against most Gram negative bacteria

USES
- Should be reserved for treatment of infections caused by multidrug-resistant strains, e.g.:
  - Methicillin-resistant *Staphylococcus aureus* (MRSA)
  - Vancomycin-resistant *Enterococcus* (VRE)

PK
- Short $t_{1/2}$ (5 hours)

ADRs
- Bone marrow suppression → anemia, leukopenia, pancytopenia, thrombocytopenia
- Peripheral neuropathy
- Optic neuritis

CHLORAMPHENICOL

MOA
- Binds reversibly to 50S subunit → inhibits binding of aminoacyl-tRNA to acceptor site

USES: Few indications due to availability of more effective and/or safer alternatives
- Last resort for meningitis caused by *H. influenzae*, *N. meningitidis*, *S. pneumoniae*
  - i.e., in a patient who is severely allergic to β-lactams

PK
- Short $t_{1/2}$ (3 hours)

ADRs
- **Gray baby syndrome** (due to developmental deficiency of glucuronyl transferase)

Tetracyclines

TETRACYCLINE, DOXYCYCLINE, MINOCYCLINE

MOA
- Bind reversibly to 30S subunit of bacterial ribosome → blocks binding of amino acid-charged tRNA to the acceptor site of the mRNA complex

SPECTRUM/USES: INTRACELLULAR organisms
- **VACUuM THe BR** (bed room) tonight
  - **V**ibrio spp.
  - **A**cne
  - **C**hlamydia (DOC)
  - **U**reaplasma urealyticum
  - **M**ycoplasma
  - **T**ularemia, **T**reponema
  - **H**elicobacter pylori (+ proton pump inhibitor + **BISMUTH SUBSALICYLATE** + **METRONIDAZOLE**)
  - **B**orelia burgdorferi (Lyme disease) – **DOXYCYCLINE** is DOC
  - **R**ickettsia (DOC)
  - **M**alaria (*Plasmodia*)

PK
- Widely distributed, including CSF

ADRs
- Gastrointestinal upset
- Photosensitivity
- Hepatotoxicity (pregnant women at greatest risk)
- Deposited in bone and teeth (gestational, childhood exposure) → suppression of bone growth (reversible with short term therapy), tooth discoloration

CONTRAINDICATIONS
- Children <8 years

DRUG INTERACTIONS
- Chelates di- and trivalent cations → absorption inhibited by Ca^{2+} (e.g. dairy, antacids), Zn^{2+}, iron salts

RESISTANCE
- Decreased accumulation (decreased uptake or expression of efflux transporter)
- Ribosomal protection protein (displaces tetracycline from target)
- Enzymatic inactivation of tetracycline

Glycylcyclines

TIGECYCLINE

MOA
- Similar mechanism as the tetracyclines, binds to the 30S subunit of the bacterial ribosome

SPECTRUM
- Gram positive
- Gram negative
- Anaerobes

USES
- Community acquired pneumonia
- Skin or subcutaneous tissue infections
- Abdominal infections

PK
- Very long $t_{1/2}$ (42 hours)

ADRs
- Diarrhea, nausea, vomiting

RESISTANCE
- Is more resistant against tetracycline efflux transporters and ribosomal protection proteins

Antimycobacterials

Antimycobacterials include drugs that are used in the prevention and/or treatment of infections caused by mycobacteria, including tuberculosis (TB), Mycobacterium avium-intracellulare complex, and leprosy.

FIRST LINE TREATMENTS

TUBERCULOSIS:
ISONIAZID
RIFAMPIN
ETHAMBUTOL
PYRAZINAMIDE
(ALL ARE HEPATOTOXIC)
STREPTOMYCIN
MOXIFLOXACIN/LEVOFLOXACIN

M. AVIUM COMPLEX-INTRACELLULARE:
AZITHROMYCIN
ETHAMBUTOL
+/- RIFABUTIN

LEPROSY:
DAPSONE
RIFAMPIN
+/- CLOFAZIMINE

ISONIAZID (INH, H)
MOA
- Prodrug → converted by mycobacterial catalase-peroxidase to active metabolite
- Inhibits synthesis of mycolic acid, a constituent of mycobacterial cell walls

USES
- DOC (single agent) for prophylaxis of tuberculosis
- DOC for treatment of tuberculosis (as part of a multidrug regimen)

PK
- Inactivated by acetylation (NAT2)
- $t_{1/2}$ varies according to NAT2 phenotype:
  - Fast acetylators: 30-90 minutes
  - Slow acetylators: 2-3 hours

ADRs
- Peripheral neuropathy (especially slow acetylators)
  - Due to vitamin B_6 deficiency → prevented by administration of pyridoxine
- Hepatotoxicity
- Lupus-like syndrome
- Inhibits P450 (CYP2C9)

CLOFAZIMINE
MOA
- Unclear; inhibits DNA replication

USE
- Leprosy

PK
- Very long $t_{1/2}$ (70 days)

ADRs
- Gastrointestinal distress
- Discoloration of the skin
- Ichthyosis, rash, pruritus

RIFAMPIN (RIF, R), RIFABUTIN
MOA
- Inhibits nucleic acid synthesis
- Binds to β subunit of bacterial DNA-dependent RNA polymerase → inhibits initiation of RNA replication

USES
- Mycobacterial infections, including:
  - Tuberculosis
  - Leprosy
  - M. avium intracellulare
- Prophylaxis for contacts of patients with meningococcal or H. influenzae meningitis
- Resistance develops quickly when used alone

PK
- Short $t_{1/2}$ (2 to 5 hours)

ADRs
- Hepatotoxicity
- Orange staining of body fluids
- With intermittent and/or high doses:
  - Hemolytic anemia, thrombocytopenia
  - Acute renal failure
  - Flu-like syndrome
- Induces P450

PYRAZINAMIDE (PZA, Z)
MOA
- Unclear; appears to target mycobacterial fatty acid synthase I gene, which is involved in mycolic acid synthesis

USE
- Tuberculosis

PK
- Moderate $t_{1/2}$ (9-10 hours)

ADRs
- Hepatotoxicity (elevated liver enzymes, jaundice, hepatic necrosis)
- Hyperuricemia, gout
- Nausea, anorexia
- Arthralgia

ETHAMBUTOL (EMB, E)
MOA
- Inhibits arabinosyltransferase, which is involved in mycobacterial cell wall synthesis

USES
- Tuberculosis
- M. avium intracellulare

PK
- Renal elimination (80% as unchanged drug)
- Short $t_{1/2}$ (2.4-4 hours)

ADRs
- Reversible optic neuritis (decreased visual acuity, defective red-green vision)
  - Dose-dependent
- Gout
- Hypersensitivity (e.g. rash, drug fever)

DAPSONE
MOA: Same as sulfonamides → inhibits bacterial folate synthesis

USES
- Prophylaxis and treatment of pneumocystis pneumonia (+ **TRIMETHOPRIM**)
- Leprosy

PK
- Moderate to very long $t_{1/2}$ (10-50 hours)

ADRs
- Hemolysis (especially in patients with G6PD deficiency)
- Methemoglobinemia (in patients with NADH dependent methemoglobin reductase deficiency)
- Anorexia, nausea, vomiting
- Infectious mononucleosis-like syndrome (rare)

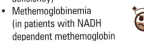

Daptomycin and Antibiotic Mnemonics

DAPTOMYCIN

MOA
- Binds to bacterial cell membrane and causes rapid depolarization, loss of membrane potential reduces DNA, RNA, and protein synthesis

SPECTRUM
- Gram positive bacteria only
- Glycoprotein-resistant enterococci
- Methicillin-resistant *Staphylococcus aureus* (MRSA)

USES
- Skin and soft tissue infections caused by Gram positive bacteria
- Bacteremia caused by *Staphylococcus aureus*

PK
- Moderate $t_{1/2}$ (8 hours)

ADRs
- Diarrhea
- Vomiting
- Pain in throat

Drugs with All Liver Metabolism
(dosage not altered for kidney failure patients)
Note: LIVE(r) is in there to remind you that these are liver metabolites

East Coast Congressional Republicans LIVE(r) Day to Day in DC
Erythromycin
Clindamycin
Chloramphenicol
Rifampin
Dicloxacillin/Cloxacillin
TMP-SMX
Dapsone
Doxycycline
Ceftriaxone

Hepatotoxic Drugs
PIES
Pyrazinomide
INH
Erythromycin
TMP-SMX

Ototoxic Drugs
VEGS
Vancomy**cin**
Erythromy**cin** (all macrolides)
Gentami**cin**
Streptomy**cin**

Bile Excretion
Dicloxacilin/Cloxacillin
Ceftriaxone
Dapsone

Antibacterials Effective Against Aerobes
GAS CC
Gentamycin
Aztreonam
SMX
Ciprofloxacin
Cefapime

Antibacterials Effective Against Intracellular Organisms
MDs **C**an **C**ure **R**are **C**onditions
Macrolides
Doxycycline
Chloramphenicol
Ciprofloxacin
Rifampin
Clindamycin

Drugs that Chelate di- and Trivalent Ions
Chloramphenicol
Chloroquine
Ciprofloxacin
Tetracycline
Antifungals (azoles)

G6PD Contraindicated
TMP/SMX	Hepatotoxic
Isoniazid	Hemolysis
Dapsone	Hemolysis

Antifungals

The Following Principles Guide the Development and Use of Antifungal Agents

- Antifungal drugs exploit biochemical differences between fungal and mammalian cells; unlike bacteria, however, fungi are also eukaryotic organisms, making it more difficult to find fungal targets that do not exist in human cells.
- Fungal cell membranes contain ergosterol, whereas mammalian cell membranes contain cholesterol.
- Fungal infections are difficult to treat because of slow growth in generally poorly vascularized areas.
- Medical advances (surgery, cancer treatment, AIDS treatment, etc.) have led to increased numbers of immunocompromised patients and an increase in opportunistic fungal infections.

Common fungal infections in the U.S. and Canada include: *Candida albicans* (most common), *Histoplasma capsulatum* (midwest-Ohio river valley), *Coccidioides immitis* ("valley fever"; dry desert areas, especially California), *Aspergillus* (immunocompromised patients), *Blastomyces* (Mississippi River valley and south-central U.S.)

The drugs are presented here according to their mechanism of action. Antifungal agents in current clinical use focus on one of four cellular targets or processes:

1. **Cell membrane integrity**
   - Form pores in the cell membrane and disrupt membrane stability and function
2. **Sterol synthesis**
   - Inhibit the synthesis of an integral part of the fungal cell membrane
3. **Nucleic acid synthesis and cell division**
4. **Glucan synthesis**
   - Inhibit fungal cell wall synthesis

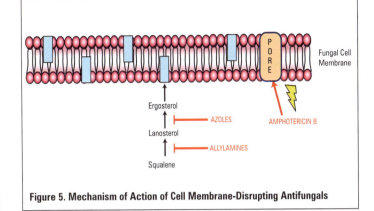

Figure 5. Mechanism of Action of Cell Membrane-Disrupting Antifungals

Class 1: Polyene Antifungals (Cell Membrane Disruptors)

AMPHOTERICIN B

MOA
- Binds ergosterol and inserts into membrane
- Facilitates pore formation → alters membrane permeability, resulting in the leakage of ions and macromolecules out of the fungal cell

USE: Broad spectrum
- DOC for life-threatening systemic fungal infections, especially in neutropenic and AIDS patients
- Intrathecal for patients with coccidiodal meningitis

PK
- Limited penetration into CNS
- Biphasic elimination:
  - Very long initial $t_{1/2}$ (24 hours)
  - Very long terminal $t_{1/2}$ (15 days)

ADRs ("Ampho-terrible" is one of the most toxic drugs in use)
- Infusion-related:
  - Fever and chills ("shake 'n' bake" syndrome)
  - Headache
  - Nausea, vomiting
  - Hypotension
  - → premedicate with acetaminophen, glucocorticoids, antihistamine and saline load
- Nephrotoxicity (renal tubular acidosis, wasting of K^+ and Mg^{2+})
  - Histological damage is permanent
  - Functional damage is usually reversible
- Hypochromic, normocytic anemia

NYSTATIN
MOA: Same as **AMPHOTERICIN B**

USES: Cutaneous or mucosal candidiasis

PK
- Minimal absorption (oral or topical)
- Excreted in the feces (following oral administration)

ADRs
- Irritation of skin, mucous membranes
- Nausea, vomiting (following oral administration)
- More toxic than **AMPHOTERICIN B** → no parenteral administration

Class 6: Echinocandins

CASPOFUNGIN

MOA
- Inhibits 1,3-β-glucan synthase
  - β-D-glucan is an integral part of the fungal cell wall

USES
- Invasive aspergillosis refractory to other antifungals
- Candidiasis

PK
- Poor oral bioavailability → IV only
- Moderate $t_{1/2}$ (9-11 hours)

ADRs
- Phlebitis (at the infusion site)
- Gastrointestinal distress (nausea, vomiting, diarrhea, abdominal pain)
- Rash, erythema
- Elevated liver enzymes
- Flushing
- Hypotension

Antifungals

Class 2: Azoles Antifungals (Cell Membrane Disruptors)

MOA
- Inhibition of lanosterol-14-α-demethylase → inhibition of ergosterol biosynthesis and accumulation of 14-α-methylated precursors
  - Altered membrane fluidity and activity of membrane-bound enzymes

SPECTRUM
- *Candida* spp.
- *Cryptococcus*
- Endemic mycoses
- *Aspergillus*

ADRs
- Nausea, vomiting
- Rash
- Hepatotoxicity (elevated liver enzymes, hepatitis (rare))
- Inhibit P450 (CYP3A4)

KETOCONAZOLE
USES
- Topical and systemic mycoses

PK
- Acidic environment needed for dissolution → absorption impaired by H_2 receptor blockers or antacids
- $t_{1/2}$ is dose-dependent
  - 90 minutes for 200 mg; 4 hours for 800 mg dose

ADRs
- Adrenal suppression, inhibition of androgen synthesis
  - Gynecomastia in males is due to suppression of androgen production

FLUCONAZOLE
USES: Systemic fungal infections
- Candidiasis
- Prophylactic therapy of fungal infections in recipients of bone marrow transplants

PK
- Water soluble – all other azoles are insoluble
- Very long $t_{1/2}$ (25-30 hours)

DRUG INTERACTIONS
- Azole with the least effect on host P450

ITRACONAZOLE
USES: MOST POTENT AZOLE
- DOC for nonmeningeal histoplasmosis and blastomycosis
- Candidiasis (oropharyngeal, esophageal)

PK
- Very long $t_{1/2}$ (21-40 hours)

ADRs
- Congestive heart failure (in patients with impaired ventricular function)
- Hypertriglyceridemia

CONTRAINDICATIONS
- Ventricular dysfunction (e.g. congestive heart failure or history of)

VORICONAZOLE
USES
- Invasive fungal infections:
  - Aspergillosis (DOC)
  - Candidiasis
- Invasive aspergillosis refractory to **AMPHOTERICIN B**

PK
- Moderate $t_{1/2}$ (6 hours)

ADRs
- Visual disturbances
- Hallucinations, toxic encephalopathy
- QT prolongation, torsades de pointes
- Renal failure (with IV route)

Class 3: Synthetic Allylamines

TERBENAFINE
MOA
- Inhibits squalene epoxidase
  - Inhibition of ergosterol synthesis (needed for cell membrane synthesis)
  - Accumulation of squalene, which is toxic to the fungal cell

USE
- Dermal mycoses (drug accumulates in skin, nails, adipose tissue)
- Tinea corporis, tinea cruris, and tinea pedis
- Onychomycosis due to dermatophytes

PK
- Very long $t_{1/2}$ (22-26 hours)

ADRs
- Minimal toxicity with topical use
- Gastrointestinal distress
- Headache
- Rash
- Taste disturbances

Inhibitors of Cell Division

Class 4: Antimetabolites

FLUCYTOSINE (5-FC)
MOA
- Prodrug → deaminated by cytosine deaminase to 5-fluorouracil (antimetabolite)
- 5-fluorouracil → → → 5-fluoro-2'-deoxyuridine-5'-monophosphate (5-FdUMP)
  - 5-FdUMP is a non-competitive inhibitor of thymidylate synthetase
- Synergistic with **AMPHOTERICIN B** → 5-FC enters through membrane tears

USES: Severe fungal infections
- Cutaneous, mucocutaneous candidiasis
- Cryptococcal meningitis (+ **AMPHOTERICIN B**)
- Mycotic pneumonias

PK
- Renal excretion
- Short $t_{1/2}$ (2.5-6 hours)

ADRs
- Dose-dependent bone marrow suppression (leukopenia, thrombocytopenia, agranulocytosis)
- Nausea, vomiting, diarrhea
- Enterocolitis
- Elevated liver enzymes

Class 5: Spindle Poison

GRISEOFULVIN
MOA
- Binds to microtubular protein → disrupts mitotic spindle and inhibits mitosis

USES
- Tinea
- Onychomycosis due to dermatophyte infection
- Systemic treatment of dermatophyte infections

PK
- Deposits in keratin-containing tissues (e.g. nails, skin, hair)
- Long $t_{1/2}$ (10-20 hours)

ADRs
- Headache
- Confusion
- Nausea, vomiting, diarrhea
- Photosensitivity
- Rash, urticaria, pruritus

DRUG INTERACTIONS
- Induces P450

Antihelminthics

Helminths (also known as worms) are multicellular organisms that can cause disease. They are divided into three different classes:
1. Cestodes (tapeworms)
2. Trematodes (fluke worms)
3. Nematodes (roundworms)

Both Trematodes (fluke worms) and Cestodes (tapeworms) are members of the phylum Platyhelminthes, which are flatworms.

Helminths infect different parts of the body, depending on the species and stage of the life cycle. Therefore, antihelminthic drugs should be chosen based on the anatomical location (e.g. restricted to intestinal lumen vs. extraintestinal), class of helminth (e.g. cestodes vs. nematodes), or stage of the helminthic life cycle (e.g. ova vs. encysted stages vs. motile adult).

In the graphic on the following page, the pharmacotherapeutics are presented adjacent to a simplified schematic of some of the parasitic helminths organized by class.

Drugs that kill intestinal parasites are not well absorbed and generally have low adverse drug reaction profiles.

Quick Comparisons

Benzimidazoles
Drugs ending in "-bendazole" share a similar mechanism of action (i.e. inhibition of microtubule formation and glucose uptake) but differ slightly in their uses.

Cestode Infections
PRAZIQUANTEL and NICLOSAMIDE are both used for cestode infections but PRAZIQUANTEL is ovicidal whereas NICLOSAMIDE is not. Therefore, use PRAZIQUANTEL.

Paralytics
PYRANTEL, IVERMECTIN, and DIETHYLCARBAMAZINE are all paralytics through inhibition of acetylcholinesterase, increased GABA release, or muscle paralysis, respectively.

Mazzotti Reaction

Treatment of filarial nematodes with IVERMECTIN or DIETHYLCARBAMAZINE can cause the Mazzotti reaction, which is an immunological response to the mass release of parasite-specific antigens from dead parasites and from endosymbiotic bacteria (*Wolbachia* spp.) that live within the parasites – not a reaction to the drug itself. It is similar to a Jarisch-Herxheimer reaction.

- Characterized by fever, headache, tachycardia, hypotension, malaise, urticaria, arthralgia, swollen lymph nodes, and peripheral edema
- Begins the day after a single antihelminthic dose; peaks on the second day
- Treat with NSAIDs, glucocorticoids, antihistamines

THIABENDAZOLE

MOA
- Similar to MEBENDAZOLE

USES
- RARELY used
- Formerly used to treat cutaneous larva migrans (creeping eruption; *Ancylostoma braziliense*)

ADRs
- Anorexia
- Vomiting
- Nausea
- Dizziness

ALBENDAZOLE

MOA
- Binds β-tubulin → inhibits microtubule polymerization
- Reduces glucose uptake
- Inhibits mitochondrial fumarate reductase
- Uncouples oxidative phosphorylation

USES
- Larval stages of tapeworms (cestodes)
    - Neurocysticercosis
    - Cystic hydatid disease (*Echinococcus* spp. + PRAZIQUANTEL if cyst leaks or ruptures)
- Nematodes
    - Cutaneous larva migrans
    - Visceral larva migrans
    - Hookworm (*Ancylostoma duodenale, Necator americanus*)
    - Pinworm (*Enterobius vermicularis*)
    - Giant roundworm (*Ascaris lumbricoides*)
    - Intestinal phase of trichinosis (*Trichinella* spp.)

PK
- Moderate to long $t_{1/2}$ (8-15 hours)

ADRs
- Gastrointestinal (abdominal pain, nausea, vomiting)
- Headache
- Dizziness
- With long term therapy:
    - Elevated liver enzymes; jaundice (rare)
    - Bone marrow suppression
- Reversible alopecia

CONTRAINDICATIONS
- Ocular cysticercosis

PRAZIQUANTEL

MOA
- Affects membrane permeability to Ca^{2+}
    - Ca^{2+} influx → tetany and spastic paralysis

USES
- Many cestodes (tapeworms)
    - Taeniasis (ingestion of *Taenia* spp. larva → intestinal infection)
    - Cysticercosis (ingestion of *Taenia solium* ova → extraintestinal infection)
        - ALBENDAZOLE preferred in neurocysticercosis
    - Diphyllobothriasis (fish tapeworm)
- Most trematodes (flatworms or flukes)
    - Schistosomiasis
    - Paragonimiasis
    - Clonorchiasis

PK
- Short $t_{1/2}$ (0.8-3 hours)

ADRs (very rapid onset)
- Gastrointestinal upset (abdominal pain, nausea, diarrhea)
- Headache, dizziness, sedation
- Better tolerated by children than adults

CONTRAINDICATIONS
- Ocular cysticercosis

Antihelminthics

MEBENDAZOLE

MOA
- Binds to β-tubulin → inhibits microtubule polymerization
- Reduces glucose uptake
- Inhibits mitochondrial fumarate reductase
- Uncouples oxidative phosphorylation

USES: Gastrointestinal nematodes (roundworms)
- Hookworm (*N. americanus, A. duodenale*)
- Pinworm (*E. vermicularis*)
- Whipworm (*Trichuris trichiura*)
- Giant roundworm (*A. lumbricoides*)
- Trichinosis (*Trichinella spiralis*)
- Active against both larval and adult stages
- Ovicidal for *Ascaris* and *Trichuris*

PK
- Short to moderate $t_{1/2}$ (3-9 hours)

ADRs
- Gastrointestinal upset
- Diarrhea
- Pruritus, rash

PYRANTEL

MOA (think organophosphate poisoning for a worm)
- Persistent activation of nicotinic acetylcholine receptors (depolarizing neuromuscular blocking agent)
  - Activates nonselective cation channels → acetylcholine release
  - Inhibits cholinesterases
- Acts on adult worms only

USES
- Enterobiasis (alternative to MEBENDAZOLE and ALBENDAZOLE)
- Hookworm

ADRs
- Transient, mild, and infrequent
- Gastrointestinal upset
- Headache
- Dizziness

IVERMECTIN

MOA
- Activates glutamate-gated Cl⁻ channels
  - Cl⁻ influx → hyperpolarization → tonic paralysis
- Also binds to GABA and other ligand-gated Cl⁻ channels

USES: Broad spectrum (nematodes, insects, mites)
- Onchocerciasis (*Onchocerca vulvulus*; river blindness)
- Strongyloidiasis

PK
- Long $t_{1/2}$ (18 hours)

ADRs
- Pruritus
- Dizziness
- Mazzotti reaction (minimal); better tolerated than DIETHYLCARBAMAZINE

DIETHYLCARBAMAZINE

MOA
- Immobilizes worm muscles → detaches scolex
- Changes worm surface membranes → host immune response susceptibility

USES
- Filariasis (*W. bancrofti, B. malayi*)
- Loiasis (*Loa loa*)

PK
- Moderate $t_{1/2}$ (8 hours)

ADRs
- Gastrointestinal (anorexia, nausea, vomiting)
- Headache
- Severe Mazzotti reaction (pretreat with glucocorticoids, antihistamines)

NICLOSAMIDE

MOA
- Inhibits glucose uptake and anaerobic metabolism
- Uncouples oxidative phosphorylation
- Kills scolex and proximal segments of the tapeworm on contact

USES
- Intestinal adult tapeworm infections
  - *Taenia* spp., *Diphyllobothrium latum*
- Not ovicidal

ADRs (rare)
- Gastrointestinal (nausea, vomiting, anorexia, diarrhea)
- Neurological (headache, drowsiness, dizziness)

NEMATODES

Wuchereria bancrofti (filariasis) *Brugia malayi* (filariasis) *Loa loa* (loiasis)	DIETHYLCARBAMAZINE
Onchocerca volvus (river blindness) *Strongyloides stercoralis* (strongyloidiasis)	IVERMECTIN
Toxocara canis (visceral larva migrans) *Ascaris lumbricoides* (ascariasis) *Ancylostoma duodenale* (hookworm) *Necator americanus* (hookworm) *Enterobius vermicularis* (pinworm) *Trichinella spiralis* (trichinosis) *Trichuris trichuria* (whipworm)	MEBENDAZOLE/ PYRANTEL

ENCYSTED LARVAL CESTODES (tissue)

Echinococcus granulosus (cystic hydatid disease) *E. multiocularis* (alveolar hydatid disease) *Taenia solium* (pork ova-cystercercosis)	ALBENDAZOLE (First line therapy)

INTESTINAL CESTODES

Taenia solium (pork larvae-taeniasis) *T. saginata* (beef larvae-taeniasis) *Diphyllobothrium latum* (fish tapeworm)	PRAZIQUANTEL

TREMATODES

Schistosoma mansoni (schistosomiasis) *S. japonicum* (schistosomiasis) *S. haemobium* (schistosomiasis) *Clonorchis sinensis* (Chinese liver fluke) *Paragonimus westermani* (lung fluke)	PRAZIQUANTEL

Antimalarials

Protozoans are unicellular organisms that infect humans at the cellular level. Generally speaking, there are two classes of protozoa: (1) blood/tissue, and (2) intestinal protozoa.

Malaria is the most significant disease caused by protozoa (*Plasmodium* spp.) and is outlined in greatest detail here. Other protozoan infections are also relevant and their treatments are discussed later. The most common intestinal protozoa in the Western World are treated with **METRONIDAZOLE**.

Malaria is the number one killer of children in Africa and is caused by five species of plasmodia.

Species	Cells infected	Note
P. falciparum	All RBCs	Many strains are resistant to **CHLOROQUINE**; can cause severe and fatal infection
P. malariae	Senescent RBCs	
P. vivax, P. ovale	Mature RBCs	Can enter into dormant stage (hypnozoites) in the liver
P. knowlesi		Simian malaria; Southeast Asia; can cause severe and fatal infection in humans

- *Plasmodium* spp. have a complex life cycle with both intracellular and extracellular components
- **Tissue schizonticides** refer to drugs that kill schizonts and hypnozoites in the liver only
- **Blood schizonticides** are drugs that kill plasmodia within erythrocytes (N.B. plasmodia within the brain or spleen are contained within erythrocytes located in capillary beds and thus are still considered intra-erythrocytic)
- **DOXYCYCLINE** kills intracellular parasites; it may be used as a single agent for prophylaxis or used in combination with a quinine-derivative or artesunate for treatment (N.B. **DOXYCYCLINE** is never used as single agent for treatment of infection)
- Malaria may be prevented by pharmacologic prophylaxis or treated in the acute setting
- **CHLOROQUINE**-resistance is becoming increasingly common; especially in the case of *P. falciparum* infections
- **ARTESUNATE** is a newer antimalarial drug in a class called *artemisinins*, derived from the sweet wormwood plant (*Artemisia annua*)
  - IV **ARTESUNATE** has been approved for use in Canada and the US as the first-line treatment for severe malaria

DOXYCYCLINE (tetracycline antibiotic)
MOA (see Antibacterials section)
- Inhibits malarial protein synthesis

USES
- Drug-resistant *P. falciparum* infections (+ **ARTESUNATE** or **QUININE**-derivative)
- Malaria prophylaxis, especially in Southeast Asia, where multidrug-resistant strains of *P. falciparum* are endemic

OTHER INFORMATION
- Please see Tetracycline Antibiotic section

ATOVAQUONE-PROGUANIL
MOA
- **ATOVAQUONE** inhibits electron transport at the cytochrome bc1 complex
- **PROGUANIL**, via metabolism to cycloguanil, inhibits dihydrofolate reductase

USES
- Malaria caused by any of the five *Plasmodium* spp.
- Prophylaxis of **CHLOROQUINE** and multi-drug resistant *P. falciparum*

PK
- Long $t_{1/2}$
  - **ATOVAQUONE**, 32 to 84 hours in adults; 24 to 48 hours in children
  - **PROGUANIL**, 12 to 21 hours

ADRs
- Cough, nausea
- Elevated liver enzymes, hepatitis (rare)
- Headache, dizziness, asthenia

CONTRAINDICATIONS
- Renal impairment
- Pregnancy

Antimalarials

PRIMAQUINE (tissue schizonticides)

MOA
- Unclear

USES
- The only antimalarial that is effective during quiescent stages in the liver (e.g. hypnozoites)
- Radical cure of *P. vivax* or *P. ovale* malaria
  - Used in conjunction with other antimalarials
- **PRIMAQUINE** anti-relapse therapy after malaria prophylaxis to prevent relapsing malaria due to *P. vivax* or *P. ovale*

PK
- Moderate $t_{1/2}$ (6 hours)

ADRs
- Abdominal pain
- Common in patients with G6PD deficiency
  - Hemolytic anemia
  - Methemoglobinemia (especially in people with nicotinamide adenine dinucleotide (NAD) methemoglobin reductase deficiency)
- Rare
  - Cardiac arrhythmia
  - Leukopenia, agranulocytosis

CONTRAINDICATIONS
- Active rheumatoid arthritis or lupus erythematosus (due to predisposition to granulocytopenia)
- Concomitant or recent use of quinacrine
- Concomitant use of other hemolytics or myelosuppressants
- Pregnancy
- Severe G6PD deficiency

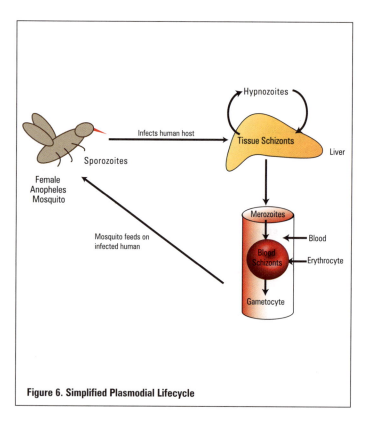

Figure 6. Simplified Plasmodial Lifecycle

CHLOROQUINE (prototypical antimalarial)

MOA
- Inhibits detoxification of heme to hemozoin
- Binds to heme from the breakdown of hemoglobin
- Heme-chloroquine complex disrupts membrane function → cell lysis

USES
- Erythrocytic forms of *P. vivax*, *P. ovale*, *P. malariae*, *P. knowlesi*, and sensitive strains of *P. falciparum*
- **Treatment and prophylaxis of malaria in pregnancy**
- Prophylaxis of *P. falciparum* in areas with known falciparum **CHLOROQUINE** susceptibility

PK
- Very long $t_{1/2}$ (3 to 5 days)

ADRs
- Pruritus (most common in dark-skinned individuals)
- With prolonged use:
  - ECG abnormalities
  - Confusion
  - Convulsions
  - Visual disturbances (keratopathy and retinopathy)

CONTRAINDICATIONS
- Retinal/visual field changes
- Seizure disorder

DRUG INTERACTIONS
- Divalent cations inhibit absorption (e.g., Ca^{2+}, Mg^{2+})

MEFLOQUINE

MOA
- Unclear; probably similar to **CHLOROQUINE**

USES
- Prophylaxis of **CHLOROQUINE**-resistant *P. falciparum* and *P. vivax*

PK
- Very long $t_{1/2}$ (20 days)

ADRs
- Neuropsychiatric:
  - Anxiety, depression
- Gastrointestinal upset
  - Bradycardia

CONTRAINDICATIONS
- Prophylaxis in patients with history of:
  - Seizure disorders
  - Serious psychiatric disorder (e.g., generalized anxiety, depression, psychosis, schizophrenia)

DRUG INTERACTIONS
- Increased risk of ECG abnormalities associated with concomitant administration of β-blockers
- Increased risk of ECG abnormalities and seizures associated with concomitant administration of **CHLOROQUINE**, **QUININE**, or **QUINIDINE**

Nonmalarial Antiprotozoals

Blood and Tissue Protozoal Infections

Chagas Disease
(*Trypanosoma cruzi*)
NIFURTIMOX

Leishmaniasis
(*Leishmania* spp.)
Antimonials such as **STIBOGLUCONATE**

African Trypanosomiasis (sleeping sickness)
(*Trypanosoma brucei gambiense, T.b. rhodesiense*)
SURAMIN (*T.b. gambiense, T.b. rhodesiense*; hemolymphatic stage)
PENTAMIDINE (*T.b. gambiense*; hemolymphatic stage)
MELARSOPROL (*T.b. gambiense, T.b. rhodesiense*; CNS involvement)

Toxoplasmosis
(*Toxoplasma gondii*)
Combination of:
TMP/SMX
PENTAMIDINE
PYRIMETHAMINE
CLINDAMYCIN
ATOVAQUONE

Babesiosis
(*Babesia microti, B. duncani, B. divergens*)
ATOVAQUONE + AZITHROMYCIN
or
QUININE + CLINDAMYCIN

Intestinal Protozoal Infections

Giardiasis (*Giardia lamblia*) **METRONIDAZOLE**

Amebiasis (*Entamoeba histolytica*; non-pathogenic sister species *E. dispar*)
METRONIDAZOLE + IODOQUINOL

Cyclosporiasis (*Cyclospora cayetanensis*) **TMP/SMX**

Cryptosporidiosis (*Cryptosporidium parvum*) nitazoxanide or paromomycin

Dientamoebiasis (*Dientamoeba fragilis*) **METRONIDAZOLE** or **IODOQUINOL**

Microsporidiosis (many species)

Also:
Protozoal vaginitis (*Trichomonas vaginalis*; infects the vagina not the intestine)
METRONIDAZOLE

> USE **METRONIDAZOLE** TO TREAT THINGS BELOW
> THE DIAPHRAGM (i.e. the intestines and vagina)
>
> **GET on the METRO**
>
> **G**iardia, **E**ntamoeba, **T**richomonas

NIFURTIMOX
MOA
- Undergoes partial reduction to nitro-anion radicals → damage, death

PK
- Short $t_{1/2}$ (3 hours)

ADRs
- Myalgia, arthralgia
- Peripheral neuropathy
- CNS (headache, paresthesias, psychological disturbances)

STIBOGLUCONATE
MOA
- Interferes with the trypanothione redox system

ADRs
- ECG abnormalities
- Pancreatitis
- Transient elevation of liver enzymes
- Bone marrow suppression
- Myalgia, arthralgia

NOTES
- Part of a class of therapeutics known as pentavalent antimonials which includes meglumine antimoniate

PYRIMETHAMINE
MOA
- Inhibits folate metabolism via inhibition of dihydrofolate reductase

PK
- Very long $t_{1/2}$ (80-95 hours)

ADRs
- Megaloblastic anemia (due to folate deficiency); blood dyscrasias

QUININE
MOA
- Similar to **CHLOROQUINE**

PK
- Moderate $t_{1/2}$ (11 hours)

ADRs
- Cinchonism
- Hypoglycemia (due to hyperinsulinemia)
- Hypotension
- Cardiac dysrhythmia
- Ototoxicity

CONTRAINDICATIONS
- Myasthenia gravis
- G6PD deficiency

METRONIDAZOLE
MOA
- Reactive intermediates react with O_2 to form superoxide anions → lipid, DNA peroxidation

USES
- Intestinal protozoal infections
- *Helicobacter pylori* infection (+ antacid + **TETRACYCLINE/AMOXICILLIN**)
- Bacterial vaginosis
- Trichomoniasis
- Rosacea

PK
- Moderate $t_{1/2}$ (8 hours)

ADRs
- Darkened urine
- Metallic taste in the mouth
- Disulfiram-like reaction (with alcohol)
- Peripheral neuropathy

IODOQUINOL
MOA
- Unclear

ADRs
- Rash, pruritus
- Enlargement of the thyroid gland
- Optic neuritis

CONTRAINDICATIONS
- Renal or hepatic impairment
- Chronic diarrhea (especially in children)
- Allergy to iodine

Autonomic Drugs

Chapter Authors: Andrew W. Browne, Sanjog Kalra, Amina I. Malik and Margaret A. Stefater

Faculty Reviewer: Lisa Thurgur

IN THIS CHAPTER

Autonomic System Overview	36
The Adrenergic System	38
The Cholinergic System	39
Glaucoma	40
Open Angle Glaucoma	
Closed Angle Glaucoma	

DRUGS IN THIS CHAPTER

Generic Name	US Trade Name	Canadian Trade Name
acebutolol	SECTRAL	RHOTRAL, SECTRAL
acetazolamide	DIAMOX	
α-methyldopa	ALDOMET	METHYLDOPA
atenolol	TENORMIN	
atracurium	TRACRIUM	
atropine	ATROPINE CARE, OCU-TROPINE, SAL-TROPINE, ATREZA	LOMOTIL
betaxolol	BETOPTIC, KERLONE	BETOPTIC
bethanecol	URECHOLINE	
bisoprolol	ZEBETA	MONOCOR
brimonidine	ALPHAGAN, COMBIGAN	
carbachol	MIOSTAT	
carteolol	CARTROL, OCUPRESS	
carvedilol	COREG	
clonidine	CATAPRES, DURACION, KAPVAY, NEXICION	CATAPRES, DIXARIT, IOPIDINE
dobutamine	DOBUTREX	
dofetilid	TIKOSYN	
donepezil	ARICEPT	
dorzolamide	TRUSOPT	COSOPT, TRUSOPT
echothiophate	PHOSPHOLINE	
edrophonium	ENLON, REVERSOL	ENLON
epinephrine	EPIPEN, PRIMATENE MIST, TWINJECT, ADRENALIN, ADRENACLICK	EPIPEN
ergotamine	ERGOMAR	BELLERGAL, CAFERGOT, ERGODRYL, GRAVERGOL, MIGRANAL
galantamine	RAZADYNE	REMINYL
guanabenz	WYTENSIN	
guanfacine	TENEX, INTUNIV	
ipratropium	ATROVENT, COMBIVENT, DUONEB	ATROVENT, COMBIVENT, DUOVENT
isoproterenol	ISUPREL	
labetalol	NORMODYNE, TRANDATE	TRANDATE
latanoprost	XALATAN	XALACOM, XALATAN
methacholine	PROVOCHOLINE	
metoprolol	TOPROL	BETALOC, LOPRESSOR
midodrine	PROMAMATINE, ORVATEN	
mirtazapine	REMERON	
modafinil	PROVIGIL	ALERTEC
naphazoline	AK-CON, ALBALON, ALLERSOL, CLEAR EYES, NAPHCON, OCU-ZOLINE, PRIVINE, VASOCLEAR	AK-CON, ALBALON, BLUE COLLYRIUM, CLEAR EYES, CIOPTICON, NAPHCON, OPCON, VISINE
neostigmine	PROSTIGMIN	
norepinephrine	LEVOPHED	
oxybutynin	OXYTROL, DITROPAN, GELNIQUE	OXYTROL, DITROPAN, UROMAX
pancuronium	PAVULON	
phenylephrine	AK-DILATE, NEOFRIN, NOSTRIL, PREFRIN, OCU-PHRIN, VICKS, SINEX, MYDFRIN	AK-DILATE, AK-VERNACON, BENYLIN, CLEAR EYES, CONTAC, DAYQUIL, DIMETAPP
pilocarpine	OCUSERT	PILOPINE, SALAGEN, TIMPILO
prazosin	MINIPRESS	
propranolol	INDERAL	
pyridostigmine	MESTINON, REGONOL	MESTINON
salbutamol	VENTOLIN	AIROMIR, COMBIVENT, VENTOLIN
scopolamine	TRANSDERM	BUSCOPAN, TRANSDERM
sotalol	BETAPACE, SORINE	
succinylcholine	QUELICIN, ANECTINE	QUELICIN
tamsulosin	FLOMAX	
terazosin	HYTRIN	
terbutaline	BRETHINE	BRICANYL TURBUHALER
timolol	TIMOPTIC, OCUDOSE, BLOCADREN, ISTALOL	TIMOPTIC
tiotropium	SPIRIVA	
varenicline	CHANTIX	CHAMPIX
vecuronium	NORCURON	
yohimbine		

Autonomic System Overview

Pharmacologic Organization of the Autonomic Nervous System

- Two divisions: sympathetic and parasympathetic that exist in balance to maintain homeostasis; BOTH are constantly active
- MOST organs are innervated by both sympathetic and parasympathetic fibers, though some exceptions exist
    - Sweat glands, adrenal medulla, erector papillae muscles, some blood vessels have ONLY SYMPATHETIC INNERVATION
- If the effects of one division are blocked or antagonized the clinical effect is that of **unopposed stimulation** of the other (e.g. β-blocker induced bradycardia occurs due to unopposed parasympathetic tone from blockade of sympathetic tone at β-receptors)
- The effect of any drug is a result of the specific receptor it binds to, the type of tissue(s) expressing the receptor, and the tissue concentration of the receptor

G-Protein Coupled Receptors

- Pharmacologic receptors are either **ionotropic** (effects via modulation of ion-channels) or **metabotropic** (effects via stimulation of "second-messenger" intracellular molecules)
- All autonomic receptors (except nAChR) are metabotropic, G-Protein Coupled Receptors (GPCRs)
- Receptor stimulation results in activation or inhibition of an intracellular enzyme that mediates downstream molecules capable of opening and closing intracellular ion channels

G-protein	Stimulatory or Inhibitory	Second Messenger	Cascade	Net Effect	Receptors
G_q	Stimulatory	PLC (increased activity)	PLC creates DAG and IP_3 from PIP_2	↑Ca^{2+}	α_1, $M_{1,3}$
G_s	Stimulatory	Adenylate Cyclase (increased activity)	Increased cAMP, PKA generation/activity	↑Ca^{2+}	β_1, β_2
G_i	Inhibitory	Adenylate Cyclase (decreased activity)	Decreased cAMP, PKA generation/activity	↓Ca^{2+}	α_2, M_2

PLC = Phospholipase C; DAG = diacyl glycerol; IP_3 = inositol-1,4,5-triphosphate;
PIP_2 = phosphatidylinositol 4,5-bisphosphate; cAMP = cyclic adenosine monophosphate;
PKA = protein kinase A

Components and Effectors of the Autonomic Nervous System Grouped by Division

	Parasympathetic Division	Sympathetic Division
Preganglionic Cell Bodies	Cranial Nerves 3,7,9,10 and sacral spine	Thoracolumbar spine (T1-L2)
Preganglionic Fiber Length	Long	Short
Preganglionic Receptors and Neurotransmitters	Nicotinic AChR (nAChR) and Acetylcholine	Nicotinic AChR (nAChR) and Acetylcholine
Postganglionic Cell Bodies	Parasympathetic ganglia (at end organs)	Sympathetic ganglia (paraspinal)
Postganglionic Fiber Length	Short	Long
Postganglionic Neurotransmitters	Acetylcholine	Norepinephrine, Epinephrine¤
End-Organ Receptors	Muscarinic AChRs (mAChR)	α_1, α_2; β_1, β_2, β_3

AChR = acetylcholine receptor

NOTES
¤ Sympathetic system uses acetylcholine at sweat glands (via mAChRs) and at the adrenal medulla (nAChRs)

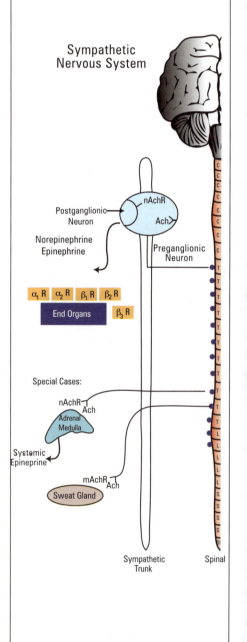

Figure 1A. Schematic of Sympathetic and Parasympathetic Nervous System

Autonomic System Overview

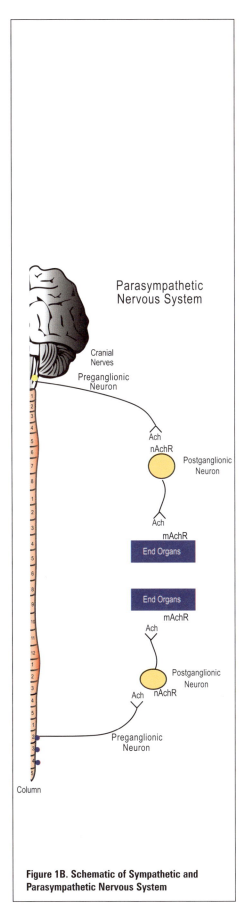

Figure 1B. Schematic of Sympathetic and Parasympathetic Nervous System

Adrenergic Stimulation
(Neurotransmitter: Norepinephrine)

Organ	Physiologic Effect	Receptor
Eye Muscles		
Radial	Contraction (mydriasis)	α_1
Sphincter	—	—
Ciliary	Relaxation (far vision)	β_2
Ocular ciliary body	Aqueous humor secretion	β_2
Major Glands		
Salivary	Amylase secretion	β_2
Nasopharyngeal	—	—
Posterior pituitary	ADH secretion	β_1
Pancreatic islet cells	Insulin secretion	β_2
Pancreatic acinar cells	Decreased secretion	α_2
Adrenal medulla	—	—
Heart		
SA Node	Increased heart rate	$\beta_1 > \beta_2$ (minor role)
AV Node	Increased conduction velocity	$\beta_1 > \beta_2$ (minor role)
Myocardium	Increased contractility	$\beta_1 > \beta_2$ (minor role)
Arterial System		
Cerebral	Vasoconstriction	α_1
Coronary	Vasoconstriction/Vasodilation	$\alpha_1/\alpha_2, \beta_2$
Pulmonary	Vasoconstriction/Vasodilation	α_1/β_2
Abdominal	Vasoconstriction/Vasodilation	α_1/β_2
Kidney	Vasoconstriction/Vasodilation	$\alpha_1, \beta_1/\beta_2$
Superficial skin, mucosa	Vasoconstriction	α_1
Skeletal muscle	Vasoconstriction/Vasodilation	α_1, β_2
Lungs		
Bronchial smooth muscle	Bronchodilation (relaxation)	β_2
Bronchial secretions	Decreased secretions	α_1 (minimal)
Stomach		
Secretions	—	—
Motility	Decreased	α_1
Intestine		
Secretions	Decreased	—
Motility	Decreased	α_1, β_2
Gallbladder	Relaxation	
Liver Exocrine Function	Gluconeogenesis/Glycogenolysis	α_1/β_2
Genitourinary System		
Kidney (Renin Release)	Inhibited/Stimulated	α_1/β_2
Bladder detrusor muscle	Inhibition of contraction	β_2
Sphincter	Contraction (stops urination)	α_1
Erection	Stimulated	α_1, α_2 (minor role)
Ejaculation	—	α_1
Skin		
Sweat glands	—	—
Erector papillae muscle	Contraction (piloerection)	α_1

Cholinergic Stimulation
(Neurotransmitter: Acetylcholine)

Organ	Physiologic Effect	Receptor
Eye Muscles		
Radial	—	—
Sphincter	Contraction (miosis)	Mainly M_3
Ciliary	Contraction (near vision)	Mainly M_3
Ocular ciliary body	—	—
Major Glands		
Salivary	Globally increased secretion	Mainly M_3
Nasopharyngeal	Globally increased secretion	Mainly M_3
Posterior pituitary	—	—
Pancreatic islet cells	Globally decreased secretion	Mainly M_3
Pancreatic acinar cells	Increased secretion	M_3
Adrenal medulla	Norepinephrine and epinephrine secretion	Nicotinic ACh
Heart		
SA Node	Decreased heart rate	M_2
AV Node	Decreased conduction velocity	M_2
Myocardium	Decreased contractility	M_2
Arterial System		
Cerebral	Vasodilation	M_3
Coronary	Vasodilation/Vasoconstriction	M_3
Pulmonary	Vasodilation (v. minimal)	M_3
Abdominal	—	—
Kidney	—	—
Superficial skin, mucosa	—	—
Skeletal muscle	Vasodilation	M_3
Lungs		
Bronchial smooth muscle	Bronchoconstriction	M_2, M_3
Bronchial secretions	Increased secretions	M_1, M_3
Stomach		
Secretions	Increased	M_3
Motility	Increased	M_3
Intestine		
Secretions	Increased	M_3
Motility	Increased	M_3
Gallbladder	Contraction	M_1, M_3
Liver Exocrine Function	—	—
Genitourinary System		
Kidney (Renin Release)	—	—
Bladder detrusor muscle	Stimulation of contraction	M_3
Sphincter	Relaxation (allows urination)	M_3
Erection	Stimulated	M_3
Ejaculation	—	—
Skin		
Sweat glands	Stimulated	M_3*
Erector papillae muscle	—	—

*Under sympathetic control

The Adrenergic System

Selected Adrenergic Agonists and Antagonists

Receptor	Selected Agonists	Agonist Effects	Selected Antagonists	Antagonist Effects
α_1	Phenylephrine	Vasoconstriction	Prazosin	Hypotension
	Midodrine	Ejaculation	Tamsulosin	Delayed ejaculation
	Ergotamine	Gluconeogenesis	Terazosin	Hypoglycemia
	Naphazoline	Pupilary dilation, far sight accommodation	Labetolol (mixed α and β)	Urinary flow augmentation
	Modafinil	Piloerection		Decreased platelet aggregation
		Urinary retention		Sedation (central effect)
α_2	Clonidine	Platelet aggregation	Mianserin	Tachycardia
	α-methyldopa	Decreased norepinephrine release	Mirtazapine	Hypertension
	Guanfacine	Sympatholytic activity	Yohimbine (historic)	Tremors
	Guanabenz	Decreased blood pressure		Cerebral excitation
				Hyperactivity
β_1	Isoproterenol	Increased myocardial contractility	Bisoprolol	Decreased myocardial O_2 demand
	Dobutamine	Increased heart rate	Metoprolol	Hypotension
	Epinephrine	Renin release	Acebutolol	Bradycardia
	Xamoterol		Atenolol	Hyperkalemia
β_2	Salbutamol	Bronchodilation	Propranolol (non-selective β_1/β_2)	Bronchoconstriction
	Isoproterenol	Vasodilation (particularly in penis)	Labetolol (non-selective β_1/β_2)	Hypotension
	Fometerol	Glycogenolysis	Sotalol (non-selective β_1/β_2)	Bradycardia
	Salmeterol	Ocular aqueous humor secretion	Timolol (non-selective β_1/β_2)	Fatigue
	Clenbuterol	Bladder relaxation and sphincter constriction	Nadolol (non-selective β_1/β_2)	Erectile dysfunction
	Levalbuterol	Uterine smooth muscle relaxation	Carvedilol (α and β blocker)	Hypoglycemia
	Terbutaline		Butaxamine (experiments, no clinical use)	Hyperkalemia
β_3	None currently approved	Increased lipolysis (brown fat)	See non-selective antagonists	See non-selective antagonists

*** List of effects IS NOT exhaustive ***

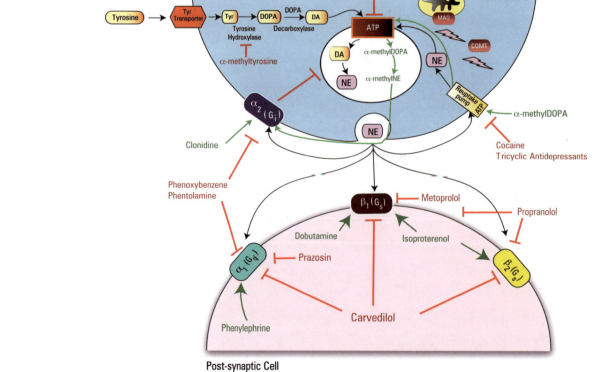

Figure 2. Schematic of an Adrenergic Synapse

The Cholinergic System

Cholinergics

These drugs cause BLUSHPADS BBC

Drug Target	Selected Agonists	Agonist Effects	Selected Uses	Contraindications

mAChR	Bethanecol
	Methacholine
	Carbachol
	Pilocarpine
		BLUSHPADS BBC
		Bradycardia
		Lacrimation
		Urination
		Salivation
		Hypotension
		Pinpoint Pupils (miosis)
		Accommodation
		Defecation (increased GI motility)
		Sweating
		Bronchoconstriction
		Bronchosecretion
		CNS dysfunction (ataxia, confusion)
			Open angle glaucoma (activates ciliary m. augmenting flow from posterior to anterior chamber; e.g. pilocarpine carbachol)
			Closed angle glaucoma (activates pupillary sphincter facilitating flow through Canal of Schlemm)
			Urinary retention (facilitates detrusor contraction and sphincter opening; e.g. bethanecol)
			Asthma testing (methacholine)
				Those who cannot tolerate :
				BLUSHPADS BBC plus
				  Peptic ulcer disease
				  Asthma
				  GI obstruction
				  Hyperthyroidism (relative)

nAChR	Nicotine
	Varenicline
	Succinylcholine
	Carbachol
		Global muscle depolarization and paralysis
		Reward behaviour
		Confusion, ataxia
			Smoking cessation (e.g. varenicline, acts as a partial nicotinic agonist for use as nicotine replacement therapy)
			Global muscle contraction, fasciculation and paralysis (e.g. succinylcholine – depolarizing paralytic agent)
				Succinylcholine contraindicated in patients with:
				  Hyperkalemia
				  Liver disease
				  Glaucoma
				  Previous malignant hyperthermia
				  Elevated CK or known myopathies

Drug Target	Selected Antagonists	Antagonist Effects	Selected Uses	Contraindications

AChE
(increases concentration of ACh in synaptic cleft by blocking the enzyme responsible for its breakdown)
	Carbamates (e.g. neostigmine, physostigmine, pyridostigmine)
	Piperidines (e.g. donepezil)
	Organophosphates (e.g. echothiophate)
	Phenanthrenes (e.g. galantamine)
	Edrophonium
		Increased parasympathetic tone, with **DUMBBELSS**:
		Diarrhea (increased GI motility)
		Urination (detrusor contraction)
		Miosis/Muscle weakness
		Bronchosecretion/Bronchospasm
		Bradycardia (and hypotension)
		Emesis
		Lacrimation
		Salivation/**S**weating
			Diagnosis of myasthenia gravis (edrophonium) and its treatment (e.g. neostigmine – intermediate acting; pyridostigmine – long acting)
			Treatment of glaucoma (e.g. physostigmine – short acting; echothiphate)
				Those who cannot tolerate BLUSHPADS BBC plus:
				  Peptic ulcer disease
				  Asthma
				  GI obstruction
				  Hyperthyroidism (relative)
				
				(Essentially same as those for cholinergic agonists)

Anticholinergics

These drugs oppose BLUSHPADS BBC

Receptor	Selected Antagonists	Antagonist Effects	Selected Uses	Contraindications
mAChR	Atropine (non-selective) Scopolamine Ipratropium, Tiotropium Oxybutynin Benztropine Mebeverine	Tachycardia Decreased GI motility (antispasmodic) Decreased bronchodilation Urinary retention Anti-parkinsonian effects Decreased bradykinesia	Emergency bradycardia reversal (atropine) IBS (scopolamine, mebeverine) COPD treatment (ipratropium, tiotropium) Bronchosecretion Overactive bladder, urge incontinence (oxybutynin) Parkinson's Disease bradykinesia (benztropine)	Narrow angle glaucoma Prostatic hypertrophy Uncontrolled tachycardia, hypertension Alzheimer's disease
nAChR	Non-depolarizing neuromuscular blockers (e.g. pancuronium, vecuronium, atracurium) Ganglionic blockers (e.g. trimethaphan)	Total paralysis via neuromuscular blockage (paralytic for surgical anesthesia) Hypotension (ganglionic nAChR blockade)	Surgical paralytic (as part of anesthesia) Blood pressure regulation (rarely)	**NEVER USED IN CONSCIOUS PATIENTS**

NOTES mAChR = Muscarinic Acetylcholine Receptor; nAChR = Nicotinic Acetylcholine Receptor; AChE = Acetylcholinesterase

Anticholinergic Toxidrome

Blind as a bat, mad as a hatter, red as a beet, hot as a hare, dry as a bone, the bowel and bladder lose their tone, and the heart runs alone.

Glaucoma

Increased intraocular pressure (IOP) from aqueous humor buildup in the eye
Normal fluid of eye (aqueous humor) is made by the ciliary body, travels through the pupil, and is drained by trabecular meshwork, at the angle of the anterior chamber.

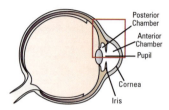
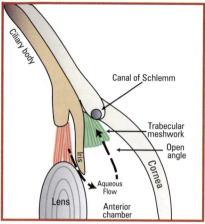
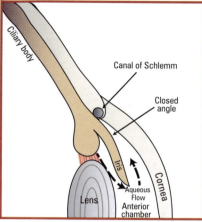

Figure 3. Anatomy of Open and Closed Angle Glaucoma

Open Angle Glaucoma

Trabecular meshwork (drainage system) not working properly
- Fluid builds up with resultant increased IOP
- Angle (between iris and cornea) of anterior chamber remains open

SYMPTOMS (slowly progressive)
- Early asymptomatic
- "Tunnel vision" (peripheral vision loss first)
- Sudden vision loss (late) due to central retinal vein occlusion
- Can progress to complete blindness

DRUGS

EPINEPHRINE
MOA
- α-agonist
- ↑ outflow of aqueous humor from posterior chamber

ADRs
- Mydriasis, stinging
- Contraindicated in closed angle!

Drugs that decrease aqueous humor production
- Prostaglandins
- Carbonic anhydrase inhibitors (see *Renal and Urological Drugs*)

Closed Angle Glaucoma

- Peripheral iris compresses the trabecular meshwork at the angle
  - Blocks aqueous humor access to trabecular meshwork
- Normal functioning trabecular meshwork, but angle is closed due to anatomical problem with iris
- Fluid cannot be drained due to blockage

SYMPTOMS (ACUTE onset)
- Sudden increase in IOP
- Red, steamy eye, severe pain
- Blurry vision (halo around light)
- Can have nonspecific symptoms (malaise, N/V, headache)
- Medical emergency! Treatment required or will result in blindness

DRUGS
Goal: cause pinpoint pupils from ↑ ACh → stretch iris → open the angle → ↑ flow
PROCHOLINERGICS
PILOCARPINE – direct cholinergic agonist
PHYSOSTIGMINE – competitive AChE inhibitor → ↑ ACh
ECHOTHIOPHATE – irreversible AChE inhibitor → ↑ ACh

ADRs
- Cyclospasm, miosis

CONTRAINDICATIONS
- Avoid dilating the pupil as this will further compress the iris and block access to the trabecular meshwork
  - α-agonists (**EPINEPHRINE**)
  - Muscarinic inhibitors (**ATROPINE, SCOPOLAMINE**)

Drugs that Work for Both Open and Closed Angle Glaucoma

1. ↓ aqueous humor synthesis
   - β-blockers → **TIMOLOL, BETAXOLOL, CARTEOLOL**
     (Tim Betta Care for glaucoma)
   - Diuretic → **ACETAZOLAMIDE, DORZOLAMIDE**
     - Inhibits carbonic anhydrase (↓HCO_3^-)
   - These drugs cause no pupillary, vision changes

2. ↑ outflow of aqueous humor
   - Prostaglandin → **LATANOPROST**
     - Darkens color of iris (**LATANOPROST** tans your iris)
   - **CHOLINOMIMETICS** (↑ endogenous ACh)
     - **PILOCARPINE, CARBACHOL, PHYSOSTIGMINE, ECHOTHIPHATE**

Pharmacology You See

Cancer Chemotherapeutics

Chapter Authors: Andrew W. Browne and Irene Zelner

Faculty Reviewers: Eric X. Chen, David J. Draper, Prateek Lala and J. Peter McPherson

IN THIS CHAPTER

Antineoplastics	42
Molecular Targeted Agents	43
Cell Cycle Specific Agents – S Phase	44
Antimetabolites	
Antitumor Antibiotics	
Topoisomerase Inhibitors	
Cell Cycle Specific Agents – M Phase	47
Plant Alkaloids	
Non-Cell Cycle Specific Agents	48
Alkylating Agents	
Platinating Agents	
Antitumor Antibiotics	
Hormonal Agents	50
Agents for Breast Cancer and Other Estrogen-Dependent Cancers	
Agents for Prostate Cancer	
Agents for Blood Cancer	

DRUGS IN THIS CHAPTER

Generic Name	US Trade Name	Canadian Trade Name
5-fluorouracil	CARAC, EFUDEX, FLUOROPLEX	EFUDEX, FLUOROPLEX
6-mercaptopurine	PURINETHOL	
anastrozole	ARIMIDEX	
bevacizumab	AVASTIN	
bleomycin	BLENOXANE	
busulfan	BUSULFEX, MYLERAN	
carboplatin		
carmustine	BICNU, GLIADEL	BICNU
cisplatin	PLATINOL	
cyclophosphamide	CYTOXAN	PROCYTOX
cytarabine	CYTOSAR-U, DEPOCYT	CYTOSAR, DEPOCYT
dactinomycin	COSMEGEN	
daunorubicin	CERUBIDINE, DAUNOXOME	CERUBIDINE
docetaxel	DOCEFREZ, TAXOTERE	TAXOTERE
doxorubicin	DOXIL	ADRIAMYCIN, CAELYX, MYOCET
erlotinib	TARCEVA	
etoposide	ETOPOPHOS	VEPESID
flutamide		EUFLEX
hydroxyurea	DROXIA, HYDREA	HYDREA
ifosfamide	IFEX	
imatinib	GLEEVEC	
leuprolide	ELIGARD, LUPRON	
methotrexate	TREXALL	METOJECT
paclitaxel	ABRAXANE, TAXOL	
prednisone		WINPRED, PREDNIDERM
rituximab	RITUXAN	
tamoxifen		NOLVADEX, TAMOX, TAMOXIFENE
topotecan	HYCAMTIN	
trastuzumab	HERCEPTIN	
vinblastine		
vincristine		

Antineoplastics

Principles of Cancer Treatment

- A single malignant cell can lead to clinically significant disease, therefore, the goal of cancer therapy is to eliminate all cancerous cells in the body
- Cancer treatment modalities: surgery, radiation, and antineoplastic agents

Cancer Chemotherapy Basics

Selectivity and Therapeutic Index
- Although antineoplastic drugs achieve some degree of selectivity by exploiting certain characteristics of cancer cells (e.g. rapid proliferation), the selectivity of most of these agents for cancer cells over normal host cells is limited, resulting in a low therapeutic index
- Doses and schedules of drug administration are often limited by normal tissue tolerance
- Effective use of antineoplastic drugs depends on the ability to balance the killing of cancer cells against the inherent toxicity of these drugs to healthy cells

The Log-Kill Hypothesis and Cyclical Therapy
- Destruction of cells by antineoplastic drugs follows first order kinetics; that is, a constant fraction of the total population of cells (e.g. 99.99%) is killed following a treatment, rather than a constant number of cells
- Sufficient cycles of treatment must be given to reduce the cancer cell burden in a proportional, stepwise manner to zero (Figure 1)
  Example: In a patient with 10^{12} cancer cells, a drug treatment that kills 99.99% of cancer cells will reduce the cancer cell burden to 10^8 after one cycle (a 4-fold log kill). Although this may induce a clinical remission, subsequent cycles are needed to eradicate the remaining (and re-growing) cells until no cancerous cells remain
- Cyclical treatment minimizes morbidity associated with toxicity as it allows for recovery of normal tissues between cycles

Combination Chemotherapy
- Advantages of combination therapy:
  - Additive or synergistic cytotoxic effect → increased cell killing
  - Suppression of drug resistance
  - Reduced toxicity to the same organ → if drugs have non-overlapping toxicities, both can be used at or near their individual maximum tolerated doses without fear of organ toxicity

Common Adverse Effects of Antineoplastic Drugs

- This section applies primarily to cytotoxic antineoplastic agents
- Many anti-cancer drugs exert their effects systemically but particularly impact rapidly dividing cells such as cancer
- Adverse effects are due to action on normal body tissues comprised of rapidly dividing cells, such as bone marrow, hair follicles, gonads, and gastrointestinal tract epithelium

MYELOSUPRESSION
- Neutropenia (most common)
  - Results in frequent infections and fever
  - Often necessitates "cycling" of therapy to allow for recovery
  - Hematopoietic colony stimulators are often used to counteract neutropenia (e.g. **FILGRASTIM**)
- Thrombocytopenia
  - Results in bleeding disorders and increased risk of hemorrhage
- Erythropoietic suppression
  - Results in anemia (may require treatment with erythropoietin)

GASTROINTESTINAL TOXICITY
- Common: anorexia, nausea, vomiting, diarrhea which can lead to:
  - Weight loss, dehydration, electrolyte imbalance, esophageal tear
- Less common: stomatitis (oral mucositis), odynophagia, esophagitis
- Often requires use of an antiemetic

DERMATOLOGIC TOXICITY
- Erythema
- Necrosis
- Alopecia (usually reversible)

GONADAL DYSFUNCTION
- Oligospermia and azoospermia
- Amenorrhea
- Usually seen with alkylating agents

SECONDARY MALIGNANCIES
- Alkylating agents → acute myelogenous leukemia (~4-5 year latency)

> **Cancer Chemotherapeutics and Pregnancy**
> Many cancer chemotherapeutics are severely teratogenic and are contraindicated in pregnancy and in patients who intend to become pregnant.

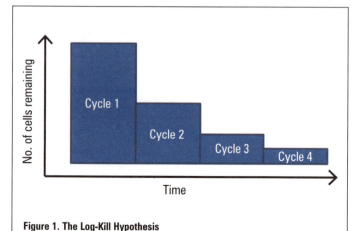

Figure 1. The Log-Kill Hypothesis

Resistance to Antineoplastic Drugs

- Cellular drug resistance is a major problem in cancer chemotherapy
- **Primary** – absence of response to drug on first exposure (the cancer cells are not susceptible to the agent)
- **Acquired** - cancer cells develop resistance to agents to which they were previously susceptible (often involves a change in gene expression)
  - Specific acquired resistance – resistance to a specific drug or a class of drugs
  - General acquired resistance - resistance to a variety of chemotherapeutic agents from different classes after exposure to a single agent
    - Example: increased expression of the *MDR1* gene that codes for a cell surface glycoprotein (P-glycoprotein) involved in drug efflux

Molecular Targeted Agents

Biologics Agents

TRASTUZUMAB

MOA
- Monoclonal antibody that binds to the human epidermal growth factor receptor 2 (HER2). HER2 mediates cell growth, differentiation and survival. HER2 receptors are overexpressed in 25-30% of primary breast cancers
- Possible mechanisms of action include down-regulation of HER2 receptors, activation of immune effector cells (antibody-dependent cell mediated cytotoxicity), reduction of S-phase cell-cycle progression, and reduction of vascular endothelial growth factor for angiogenesis

USES
- Breast cancer (HER2-positive)

PK
- Very long $t_{1/2}$ (1-32 days)

ADRs
- Cardiovascular effects: edema, cardiomyopathy, congestive heart failure
- Respiratory toxicity: cough, dyspnea, pharyngitis, pulmonary toxicity, respiratory failure
- Gastrointestinal: abdominal pain, diarrhea, nausea and vomiting
- Hepatotoxicity
- Hypersensitivity reaction
- Nephrotic syndrome (rare)
- Infusion-related syndrome: fever and chills may occur in 40% of patients during the first infusion
- Neurologic effects: asthenia, headache

BEVACIZUMAB

MOA
- Monoclonal antibody that selectively binds to and neutralizes the human vascular endothelial growth factor (VEGF). This reduces angiogenesis, thereby inhibiting tumor growth

USES
- Colorectal cancer, breast cancer (HER2-negative), lung cancer (non-small cell), glioblastoma multiforme of brain
- Intraocular injection for diseases involving ophthalmic neovascularization (e.g. diabetic retinopathy)

PK
- Very long $t_{1/2}$ (19-20 days)

ADRs
- Gastrointestinal toxicity: abdominal pain, diarrhea, loss of appetite, stomatitis, gastrointestinal perforation, tracheoesophageal fistula
- Asthenia
- Wound healing complications
- Respiratory toxicity
- Proteinuria
- Fistula of bile duct
- Hypersensitivity reaction
- Cardiovascular toxicity
- Neurologic toxicity

RITUXIMAB

MOA
- Monoclonal antibody to B-lymphocyte CD20 surface antigen

USES
- Lymphoma, chronic lymphocytic leukemia, severe rheumatoid arthritis

ADRs
- Fever, chills, body aches

Tyrosine Kinase Inhibitors

Most effective against cancers that are highly dependent upon a single protein for continued growth.

IMATINIB

MOA
- Selective inhibitor of the BCR-ABL tyrosine kinase, a fusion protein product of the Philadelphia chromosome, that is expressed in chronic myeloid leukemia. IMATINIB binds to the BCR-ABL fusion protein and impedes the tyrosine kinase activity, thereby blocking oncogenic signals
- Inhibits the receptor tyrosine kinase activity of c-kit (stem-cell factor receptor) that is constitutively active in gastrointestinal stromal tumors
- Cells that express these proteins undergo growth inhibition or apoptosis but normal cells are not affected

USES
- Chronic myeloid leukemia, gastrointestinal stromal tumors (GIST)

PK
- Long $t_{1/2}$ (13-18 hours)

ADRs
- Myelosuppression
- Cardiovascular effects: edema, congestive heart failure, chest pain, cardiogenic shock
- Dermatologic toxicity: alopecia, pruritus, rash
- Hypokalemia
- Gastrointestinal toxicity: abdominal pain, diarrhea, nausea and vomiting
- Arthralgia, myalgia
- Asthenia
- Respiratory toxicity: cough, dyspnea, pneumonia
- Fever
- Elevated billirubin, ALT, AST, alkaline phosphate

ERLOTINIB

MOA
- Epidermal growth factor receptor (EGFR) tyrosine kinase inhibitor. By inhibiting EGFR autophosphorylation, it inhibits EGF-dependent cell proliferation
- Blocks cell-cycle progression in the G1 phase

USES
- Non-small cell lung cancer, pancreatic cancer

PK
- Very long $t_{1/2}$ (36 hours)

ADRs
- INR elevations, bleeding events
- Fatigue
- Rash
- Gastrointestinal toxicity: anorexia, diarrhea, GI hemorrhage
- Increases in liver transaminases
- Interstitial lung disease
- Hepato-renal syndrome

NOTES
- GEFITINIB, and the biologics CETUXIMAB and PANITUMUMAB also target EGFR

Cell Cycle Specific Agents – S Phase

Antimetabolites

The Cell Cycle and Chemotherapeutics

- Major classes of antineoplastic agents can be categorized according to their cell cycle specificity:

Cell Cycle Specific Drugs
- Exert their effects exclusively or primarily during specific phases of the cell cycle
- Frequently ineffective against non-cycling cells (in G_0-phase)
- Most effective in hematological malignancies and tumors in which a relatively large proportion of cells are proliferating (high growth fraction)

Cell Cycle NON-specific Drugs
- Exert their effects in all phases of the cell cycle, including G_0 (cycling cells may be more sensitive)
- Useful in low growth fraction solid tumors, as well as high growth fraction tumors
- In general, cells in the active part of the cycle are most sensitive to chemotherapeutic agents, and slow growing tumors with fewer cycling cells (in G_0 phase) are relatively resistant to antineoplastic drugs

---

- Antimetabolites are structural analogues of naturally-occurring compounds, and typically act by interfering with nucleic acid or nucleotide synthesis
- These agents are most active against cells proceeding through S phase, therefore, neoplastic cells display increased susceptibility to actions of antimetabolites
- The following agents fall under this category; **METHOTREXATE, 5-FLUOROURACIL, 6-MERCAPTOPURINE** and **CYTARABINE**

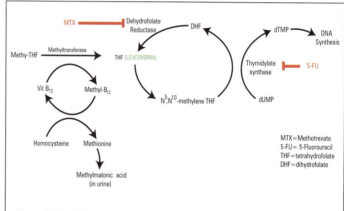

Figure 3. The Effects of MTX and 5-FU in Nucleic Acid Synthesis

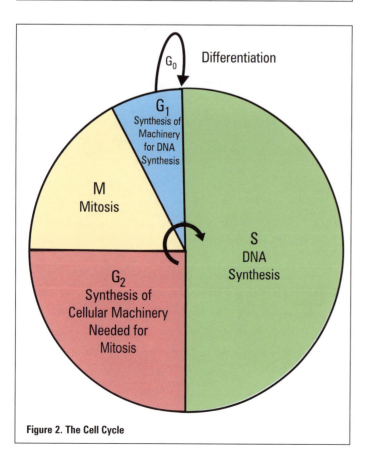

Figure 2. The Cell Cycle

METHOTREXATE (MTX)

MOA
- MTX is a folic acid antagonist. It inhibits dihydrofolate reductase (DHFR), which reduces dihydrofolates to tetrahydrofolates. This inhibition interferes with the synthesis of purine nucleotides and thymidylate, thus interfering with DNA synthesis, repair, and replication

USES
- Leukemia (acute meningeal, lymphoblastic, and lymphocytic), lymphoma (Burkitt's, childhood, non-Hodgkin's), sarcomas (lymphatic and osteogenic), choriocarcinoma, breast and bladder cancer, gastric cancer, lung cancer, head and neck cancers, leptomeningeal cancer, mycosis fungoides

PK
- Moderate to long $t_{1/2}$ (3-15 hours)

ADRs
- Severe myelosuppression
- Gastrointestinal toxicity: diarrhea, loss of appetite, nausea and vomiting, stomatitis
- Hepatotoxicity: liver failure, atrophy, necrosis, cirrhosis, fibrosis
- Nephrotoxicity (minimized by hydration).
- Neurotoxicities (with intrathecal administration or high-doses)
- Acute neurologic syndrome
- Pulmonary toxicity: acute and chronic, interstitial pneumonia
- Dermatologic toxicity: alopecia, photosensitivity, rash

Cell Cycle Specific Agents – S Phase

Antimetabolites

5-FLUOROURACIL (5-FU)

MOA
- 5-FU is a fluorinated pyrimidine analogue. It is a prodrug that undergoes a complex series of biotransformations to several ribosyl and deoxyribosyl nucleotide metabolites (FdUMP, FdUTP, FUTP) that ultimately interfere with DNA synthesis and RNA processing

USES
- Colorectal, bladder, breast, gastric, pancreatic, prostate, and head and neck cancers. Also used for actinic keratoses and skin cancer (topically)

PK
- Crosses the BBB
- Very short $t_{1/2}$ (6-22 minutes for parent drug, 50 minutes for metabolites)

ADRs
- Dermatologic toxicity: alopecia, palmar-plantar erythrodysesthesia, maculopapular eruption, photosensitivity
- Gastrointestinal toxicity: diarrhea, esophagopharyngitis, anorexia, nausea and vomiting, stomatitis, ulcer
- Cardiovascular toxicity: angina, coronary arteriosclerosis, thrombophlebitis
- Myelosuppression
- Cerebellar syndrome
- Ophthalmic toxicity

CONTRAINDICATIONS
- Bone marrow depression
- DPD enzyme deficiency (topical route)
- Poor nutritional state
- Serious infection

6-MERCAPTOPURINE (6-MP)

MOA
- 6-MP is a thiopurine analogue. It is a prodrug transformed intracellularly by the enzyme hypoxanthine-guanine phosphoribosyltransferase (HGPRT) to several active nucleotide metabolites which can interfere with various metabolic reactions necessary for RNA and DNA biosynthesis

USES
- Acute lymphocytic leukemia, acute myelogenous leukemia, and chronic myeloid leukemia

PK
- Short $t_{1/2}$ (21-90 minutes, active metabolites persist longer)

ADRs
- Dermatologic effects: hyperpigmentation of skin, rash
- Gastrointestinal toxicity: diarrhea, nausea and vomiting, stomatitis, ulcer
- Hyperuricemia
- Myelosuppression
- Hepatotoxicity

CONTRAINDICATIONS
- Concomitant use of **FEBUXOSTAT**
- Concomitant administration of live vaccines

NOTES
- Patients deficient in the detoxifying enzyme, thiopurine methyltransferase (TPMT), are more likely to develop dangerous myelosuppression
- Testing for TPMT genotype is available

CYTARABINE (ARA-C)

MOA
- Cytarabine is a synthetic pyrimidine nucleoside that is converted intracellularly to active cytarabine triphosphate (AraCTP). It inhibits DNA polymerase resulting in the inhibition of DNA synthesis. Incorporates into DNA and RNA leading to chain termination

USES
- Hematologic malignancies (acute lymphocytic and myeloid leukemia, chronic myelogenous leukemia, meningeal leukemia, non-Hodgkins lymphoma)

PK
- Short $t_{1/2}$ (1-3 hours)

ADRs
- Severe myelosuppression
- Cardiovascular toxicity: thrombophlebitis
- Rash
- Gastrointestinal toxicity: anal inflammation, diarrhea, anorexia, nausea and vomiting, stomatitis, bowel necrosis, necrotizing colitis including oral and anal ulcerations, and pneumatosis cystoides intestinalis leading to peritonitis
- Hyperuricemia
- Decreased liver function
- Infections and sepsis
- Neuropathy
- Kidney disease
- Anaphylaxis

Cell Cycle Specific Agents – S Phase

Antitumor Antibiotics

BLEOMYCIN
- Consists of a mixture of glycopeptides derived from fungal culture

MOA
- Produces DNA strand breaks through formation of an intermediate bleomycin-metal complex and intercalation into DNA. The bleomycin-metal complex may catalyze formation of reactive oxygen species which further damage DNA

USES
- Cancer of larynx, paralarynx, and nasopharynx, Hodgkin's disease, non-Hodgkin's lymphoma, malignant pleural effusion, penile cancer, renal cancer, soft tissue sarcoma, testicular cancer, vulval cancer, lung cancer, cervical cancer, head and neck cancers

PK
- Short $t_{1/2}$ (2-4 hours)

ADRs
- Respiratory toxicity: pneumonitis, interstitial pulmonary fibrosis
- Dermatologic toxicity: alopecia, erythema, rash, hyperpigmentation, skin tenderness
- Gastrointestinal toxicity: nausea, vomiting, stomatitis
- Confusion
- Hepatotoxicity
- Nephrotoxicity
- Cardiovascular effects: hypotension, myocardial infarction, vascular disorder

NOTES
- Little myelosuppression, therefore bleomycin is useful in combination therapy

HYDROXYUREA

MOA
- Inhibits ribonucleotide reductase, thereby preventing conversion of ribonucleotides to deoxyribonucleotides. Also, it inhibits the incorporation of thymidine into DNA, and may directly damage DNA

USES
- Head and neck cancer, chronic myeloid leukemia, melanoma, ovarian cancer

PK
- Crosses BBB
- Short $t_{1/2}$ (3-4 hours)

ADRs
- Myelosuppression
- Dermatologic toxicity: Gangrenous disorder, skin ulcer

CONTRAINDICATIONS
- Patients with severe bone marrow depression

Topoisomerase Inhibitors

Epipodophyllotoxins and Camptothecins

- DNA topoisomerases I and II are enzymes that relieve torsional strain of the supercoiled DNA helices during the processes of replication, transcription, and repair by forming nicks in the strands. This allows the DNA to swivel at the nicks and it is subsequently re-ligated.
- **Epipodophyllotoxins** and **Camptothecins** are topoisomerase inhibitors that bind and stabilize DNA/topoisomerase complexes thereby preventing re-ligation. This ultimately leads to DNA breaks when the replication fork encounters these complexes.

Epipodophyllotoxins

ETOPOSIDE
- A semisynthetic derivative of the podophyllotoxins (from the mandrake plant)

MOA
- Inhibits DNA topoisomerase II, leading to DNA strand breakage and cell death

USES
- Lung cancer, lymphomas, testicular cancer

PK
- Short to moderate $t_{1/2}$ (3-12 hours)

ADRs
- Hypersensitivity reaction during/soon after IV administration
- Myelosuppression
- Fatigue
- Dermatologic toxicity: alopecia, Stevens-Johnson syndrome, toxic epidermal necrolysis
- Hepatotoxicity
- Asthenia
- Gastrointestinal toxicity: anorexia, nausea and vomiting, diarrhea, stomatitis
- Cardiotoxicity: congestive heart failure, myocardial infarction

Camptothecins

TOPOTECAN
- A semisynthetic derivative of camptothecin, a cytotoxic alkaloid extracted from plants such as *Camptotheca acuminata*

MOA
- Inhibits the action of topoisomerase I leading to DNA breakage and cell death

USES
- Ovarian cancer, small-cell lung cancer, cervical carcinoma

PK
- Short $t_{1/2}$ (2-3 hours)

ADRs
- Myelosuppression
- Alopecia
- Gastrointestinal toxicity: nausea and vomiting, diarrhea
- Dyspnea

Cell Cycle Specific Agents – M Phase

Plant Alkaloids

Vinca Alkaloids

VINCRISTINE, VINBLASTINE
- Derived from the periwinkle plant, *Vinca rosea*
- Despite identical mechanism of action, they have different PK, indications, and toxicities

MOA
- Inhibit tubulin **polymerization** thereby disrupting assembly of microtubules. This results in mitotic arrest at metaphase ultimately leading to cell death

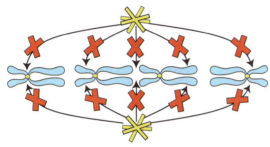

Figure 4. Mechanism of Action of Vinca Alkaloids

VINCRISTINE

USES
- Acute leukemia, Hodgkin's disease, non-Hodgkin's lymphoma, multiple myeloma, Ewing's sarcoma, Wilms' tumor, colorectal cancer, breast, cervical and ovarian cancer, neuroblastoma, small-cell lung cancer, rhabdomyosarcoma

PK
- Extensive hepatic metabolism (cytochrome P450)
- Long $t_{1/2}$ (14-25 hours)

ADRs
- Neurotoxicity – peripheral neuropathy
- Paralytic illeus

VINBLASTINE

USES
- Hodgkin's disease, non-Hodgkins lymphoma, germ cell tumor, testicular cancer, Kaposi's sarcoma, breast cancer, choriocarcinoma, mycosis fungoides

PK
- Extensive hepatic metabolism (cytochrome P450)
- Long $t_{1/2}$ (25 hours)

ADRs
- Myelosuppression – primarily leukopenia

Taxanes

PACLITAXEL, DOCETAXEL
- Plant alkaloids derived from the bark of the Pacific yew tree (*Taxus brevifolia*) and needles of the European yew tree (*Taxus baccula*), respectively

MOA
- Inhibit microtubule **depolymerization** thus disrupting the normal growth and breakdown of microtubules needed for mitosis and cell division

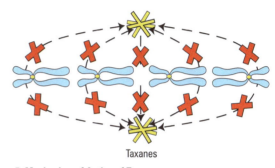

Figure 5. Mechanism of Action of Taxanes

PACLITAXEL

USES
- Breast cancer, non small-cell lung cancer, ovarian cancer, Kaposi's sarcoma

PK
- Extensive hepatic metabolism (cytochrome P450)
- Very long $t_{1/2}$ (13-52 hours)

ADRs
- Myelosuppression
- Hypersensitivity reaction – prevented with prophylactic treatment with corticosteroids and histamine antagonists
- Alopecia
- Gastrointestinal toxicity: intestinal obstruction, nausea and vomiting, diarrhea, perforation
- Infection, sepsis
- Peripheral neuropathy
- Arthralgia, myalgia
- Pulmonary embolism

DOCETAXEL

USES
- Breast cancer, non small-cell lung cancer, prostate cancer, head and neck cancers, gastric cancer

PK
- Extensive hepatic metabolism (cytochrome P450)
- Moderate $t_{1/2}$ (11 hours)

ADRs
- Myelosuppression
- Cardiovascular effects: edema, vasodilation
- Fever
- Dermatologic toxicity: alopecia, pruritus, rash, nail changes, Stevens-Johnson syndrome, toxic epidermal necrolysis
- Gastrointestinal toxicity: stomatitis, nausea and vomiting, diarrhea, colitis
- Neurologic: asthenia, neuropathy
- Amenorrhea
- Hepatotoxicity
- Renal failure
- Infection

Non-Cell Cycle Specific Agents

Alkylating Agents

MOA
- Chemically diverse drugs that act by transferring their alkyl groups to various intracellular macromolecules (e.g. DNA, RNA, proteins)
- Majority of alkylating agents are bifunctional since they have two reactive groups
- Interaction can occur on one or both strands of DNA through cross-linking. Cross-linking of DNA is a major mode of cytotoxic action
- Major site of alkylation within DNA is the N7 position of guanine. Alkylation of guanine can lead to miscoding due to abnormal base pairing with thymine or in depurination that results in DNA breakage
- Although alkylating agents are not cell cycle specific, cells are most susceptible to alkylation-induced damage in late G1 and S phases

OTHER INFORMATION
- Resistance to alkylating agents can be due to increased capability to repair DNA lesions, decreased permeability of the cell to these agents, and increased production of glutathione, which inactivates these agents via conjugation
- Agents that fall under this class include the nitrosoureas, alkyl sulfonates, and nitrogen mustards
- Alkylating agents are themselves considered carcinogenic

Alkyl Sulfonates

BUSULFAN
USES
- Conditioning regimen prior to bone marrow transplant, chronic myeloid leukemia

PK
- Crosses BBB
- Short $t_{1/2}$ (2.3-2.6 hours)

ADRs
- Cardiovascular effects and toxicity
- Pruritus, rash
- Endocrine disorders
- Nausea and vomiting, stomatitis
- Cough, dyspnea, epistaxis, rhinitis
- Neurologic effects: dizziness, insomnia, seizure
- Anxiety, depression
- Profound myelosuppression
- Veno-occlusive disease of the liver
- Hemorrhagic cystitis
- Amenorrhea, male infertility
- Pulmonary fibrosis

Nitrosoureas

CARMUSTINE
USES
- Brain tumors, non-Hodgkin's lymphoma, Hodgkin's disease, multiple myeloma

PK
- Crosses BBB
- Very short $t_{1/2}$ (<1 hour)

ADRs
- Myelosuppression
- Nausea and vomiting
- Pulmonary toxicity, infiltrates, interstitial fibrosis
- Renal toxicity
- Infection
- Decreased liver function
- Secondary malignancy

Nitrogen Mustards

CYCLOPHOSPHAMIDE, IFOSFAMIDE
USES
- Leukemia (acute and chronic myeloid and lymphoid), lymphomas, lung cancer, breast cancer, neuroblastoma, retinoblastoma, ovarian cancer, multiple myeloma, soft tissue sarcoma, mycosis fungoides

PK
- Moderate $t_{1/2}$ (3-15 hours)

NOTES
- Both agents are prodrugs that require biotransformation to active metabolites
- See also Immune Response Modifiers chapter

CYCLOPHOSPHAMIDE
ADRs
- Myelosuppression
- Cardiomyopathy
- Nausea and vomiting
- Hemorrhagic cystisis – proper hydration important
  - Note: prophylaxed with Mesna (2-mercapto ethane sulfonate sodium)
- Reproductive toxicity: amenorrhea, azoospermia, oligozoospermia
- Alopecia
- Interstitial pneumonia
- Infection
- Secondary malignancy

IFOSFAMIDE
ADRs
- Myelosuppression
- Nausea and vomiting
- Alopecia
- Neurotoxicity
- Metabolic acidosis
- Hemorrhagic cystisis – proper hydration important
  - Note: prophylaxed with Mesna (2-mercapto ethane sulfonate sodium)

Platinating Agents

CISPLATIN and CARBOPLATIN
MOA
- These agents undergo intracellular activation to form reactive platinum complexes which are believed to react with the nucleophilic sites on DNA leading to intra-strand and inter-strand cross-links

CISPLATIN
USES
- Bladder cancer, ovarian cancer, testicular cancer

PK
- Very long $t_{1/2}$ (16-53 hours)

ADRs
- Ototoxicity
- Myelosuppression
- Hypersensitivity reaction
- Neurotoxicity: cerebral herniation, encephalopathy, seizure
- Nausea and vomiting
- Nephrotoxicity

CARBOPLATIN
USES
- Ovarian cancer, brain tumors, head and neck cancers

PK
- Crosses the BBB
- Short $t_{1/2}$ (1-6 hours)

ADRs
- Myelosuppression
- Nausea and vomiting
- Electrolyte imbalance
- Hypersensitivity reaction
- Peripheral neuropathy
- Visual disturbance (rare)

Non-Cell Cycle Specific Agents

Antitumor Antibiotics

DACTINOMYCIN
- Antineoplastic antibiotic derived from *Streptomyces parvullus*

MOA
- Exerts its cytotoxic effects by binding tightly to DNA through intercalation between base pair and inhibiting DNA-dependent RNA synthesis

USES
- Gestational trophoblastic tumor, rhabdomyosarcoma, Wilms' tumor, Ewing's sarcoma, metastatic malignant tumor of testis, nephroblastoma

PK
- Very long $t_{1/2}$ (36 hours)

ADRs
- Myelosuppression
- Nausea and vomiting
- Dermatologic effects: acne, alopecia, erythema, rash
- Gastrointestinal toxicity: diarrhea, nausea and vomiting, stomatitis
- Fever
- Anaphylaxis
- Hepatotoxicity, liver failure, veno-occlusive disease of the liver

MITOMYCIN C
- Antineoplastic antibiotic isolated from *Streptomyces caespitosus*

MOA
- Undergoes biotransformation to generate an alkylating agent that causes cross-linking of DNA. It is cell cycle phase-nonspecific, although it has maximum effect in late G- and early S-phases

USES
- Pancreatic and gastric cancers, bladder cancer, colon cancer

PK
- Very short $t_{1/2}$ (23-78 minutes)

ADRs – Very toxic
- Myelosuppression
- Gastrointestinal toxicity: mucositis, nausea and vomiting, stomatitis
- Veno-occlusive renal disease
- Renal irritation
- Congestive heart failure
- Edema
- Skin photosensitivity
- Hemolytic uremic syndrome

Anthracyclines

DAUNORUBICIN, DOXORUBICIN
- Anthracycline antibiotics were isolated from *Streptomyces peucetius var caesius*

MOA
- Exert their cytotoxic effects by binding directly to DNA via intercalation between base pairs and by inhibiting topoisomerase II. This leads to blockade of DNA and RNA synthesis and DNA fragmentation. Additionally, these agents complex with iron and produce free radicals that damage DNA and cell membranes
- Although maximally cytotoxic in S phase, these agents are toxic in all phases of the cell cycle

DAUNORUBICIN
USES
- Leukemia (acute and chronic myeloid, acute lymphoid), non-Hodgkin's lymphoma, lymphosarcoma

PK
- Long $t_{1/2}$ (14-20 hours)

ADRs
- Myelosuppression
- Cardiotoxicity: congestive heart failure, dilated cardiomyopathy
- Mucositis
- Gastrointestinal toxicity: nausea and vomiting, stomatitis
- Alopecia
- Hyperuricemia

DOXORUBICIN
USES
- Non-Hodgkin's lymphoma, lymphosarcoma, bladder cancer, breast cancer, lung cancer, gastric cancer, gynecological carcinoma, head and neck cancer, hepatic carcinoma, testicular cancer, thyroid cancer, embryonal rhabdomyosarcoma, Ewing's sarcoma, Hodgkin's disease, islet cell carcinoma, Kaposi's sarcoma, neuroblastoma, osteogenic sarcoma, retinoblastoma, sarcomas, Wilms' tumor, leukemia (acute lymphoid and myeloid)

PK
- Very long $t_{1/2}$ (20-48 hours)

ADRs
- Myelosuppression
- Cardiotoxicity: arrhythmia, congestive heart failure, dilated cardiomyopathy
- Mucositis
- Gastrointestinal toxicity: nausea and vomiting, stomatitis
- Alopecia
- Hyperpigmentation
- Dysuria

Hormonal Agents

- Sex hormones stimulate and control proliferation and function of certain tissues (e.g. mammary and prostate glands, endometrium), and thus cancers arising in these tissues may be inhibited or stimulated by changes in hormone balance
- Adrenal corticosteroids (e.g. glucocorticoid analogues) have been useful in treatment of acute leukemia, lymphomas, and other hematologic cancers. These steroids cause dissolution of lymphocytes, regression of lymph nodes, and inhibition of growth of certain mesenchymal tissues

- Agents that fall under this class include the antiestrogens, antiandrogens, gonadotropin-releasing hormone agonists, and aromatase inhibitors
- Resistance to these agents can develop due to receptor down-regulation or mutations in drug targets
- These drugs have a different adverse effect profile from other antineoplastics and typically do not cause severe myelosuppression

Agents for Breast Cancer and Other Estrogen-Dependent Cancers

Aromatase Inhibitors

ANASTROZOLE

MOA
- Reversible, nonsteroidal aromatase inhibitor (see Endocrine Drugs chapter)
- Aromatase catalyzes the final step in the conversion of androgens to estrogens in peripheral tissues. By inhibiting aromatase, **ANASTROZOLE** deprives estrogen sensitive cancer cells of estrogens, thus preventing development or progression of tumors
- Does not interfere with the production of other steroids (e.g. adrenal corticosteroids, aldosterone) or thyroid stimulating hormone

USES
- Breast cancer (postmenopausal women)

PK
- Very long $t_{1/2}$ (50 hours)

ADRs
- Cardiovascular effects: peripheral edema, hypertension, chest pain, myocardial infarction, thrombophlebitis
- Dermatologic toxicity: alopecia, pruritus, rash
- Gastrointestinal toxicity: abdominal pain, nausea, diarrhea
- Hot flashes
- Hypercholesterolemia
- Fractures, osteoporosis
- Arthralgia, myalgia
- Headache
- Vaginal dryness

Selective Estrogen Receptor Modifiers (SERMs)

TAMOXIFEN

MOA
- Acts as a competitive partial agonist inhibitor of estrogen. It binds to estrogen receptors on estrogen-sensitive cancer cells, which has cytostatic effects
- Has effects independent of estrogen receptor expression that include inhibition of key enzymes and modulation of growth factor secretion
- Acts as an estrogen agonist in several tissues including endometrium, bone and lipids

USES
- Breast cancer, endometrial cancer

PK
- Undergoes extensive enterohepatic circulation
- Very long $t_{1/2}$ (5-14 days)

ADRs
- Thromboembolic events
- Sweating, hot flashes
- Vaginal bleeding
- Altered lipid profile; decreased total and LDL cholesterol, decreased HDL cholesterol, hypercholestremia, increased triglycerides
- Depression
- Cataracts
- Arthralgia/myalgia
- Secondary malignancies – endometrial cancer, uterine sarcoma
- Tumor flare syndrome

Hormonal Agents

Agents for Prostate Cancer

Gonadotropin-Releasing Hormone Agonists

LEUPROLIDE

MOA
- Potent gonadotropin releasing hormone (GnRH) analogue. It initially stimulates the release of luteinizing hormone (LH), followed by inhibition with chronic administration. This leads to a reduction in sex hormone released in response to LH stimulation
- In men, reduces serum androgen

USES
- Prostate cancer

PK
- Short $t_{1/2}$ (3 hours)

ADRs
- Drug-induced disease flare: during the initial weeks of treatment, **LEUPROLIDE** may cause a worsening (flare) of the symptoms of prostate or breast cancer – minimized with **FLUTAMIDE** (antiandrogen)
- Anemia
- Cardiotoxicity: myocardial infarction, sudden cardiac death
- Weight gain
- Hot flashes
- Decreased bone mineral density, fracture
- Decreased muscle mass
- Depression
- Memory loss
- Decreased libido

Antiandrogens

FLUTAMIDE

MOA
- Nonsteroidal antiandrogen which inhibits androgen uptake and the binding of androgens to the androgen receptor

USES
- Prostate cancer

PK
- Moderate $t_{1/2}$ (7.8 hours)

ADR
- Diarrhea, nausea
- Hot sweats
- Rash
- Hepatotoxicity, liver failure
- Myelosuppression
- Impotence

Agents for Blood Cancer

PREDNISONE
- A synthetic glucocorticoid analog. Mainly used for its anti-inflammatory effects but also has profound and varied metabolic effects. It is used in hematologic cancers

NOTES
- **PREDNISONE** immunosupressive effect on T-cells is particularly useful for lymphocytic malignancies
- See also Endocrine Drugs and Immune Response Modifiers chapters

Cardiovascular Drugs

Chapter Authors: Brian G. Ballios, Andrew W. Browne, Janine R. Hutson, James A. Stefater and Margaret A. Stefater

Faculty Reviewers: Paul Dorian and Prateek Lala

IN THIS CHAPTER

Cardiovascular Electrophysiology	55
Antiarrhythmics	56
Shock	60
Vasodilators and Vasoconstrictors	61
Nitrovasodilators	62
Sympatholytic/Anti-Adrenergic Drugs	63
Non-Autonomic Vasodilators	65
Heart Failure	67
Introduction	
Negative Inotropes	
Positive Inotropes	
Cardiac Glycosides	
Antihyperlipidemia Drugs	71

DRUGS IN THIS CHAPTER

Generic Name	US Trade Name	Canadian Trade Name
adenosine	ADENOCARD, ADENOSCAN	ADENOCARD
amiodarone	CORDARONE, PACERONE	CORDARONE
amlodipine	NORVASC	
amyl nitrite		
atenolol	TENORMIN	
atorvastatin	LIPITOR	LIPITOR, CADUET
bretylium		BRETYLIUM TOSYLATE INJECTION USP
carvedilol	COREG	
cholestyramine	PREVALITE, QUESTRAN (LIGHT)	CHOLESTYRAMINE
clofibrate	ATROMID-S	
clonidine	CATAPRES, DURACION, KAPVAY, NEXICION	CATAPRES, DIXARIT, IOPIDINE
colestipol	COLESTID	
diazoxide	HYPERSTAT, PROGLYCEM	PROGLYCEM
digoxin	DIGITEK, LANOXIN, LANOXICAPS	LANOXIN
diltiazem	CARDIAZEM, CARTIA, DILACOR, TIAZAC	CARDIAZEM, TIZAC
disopyramide	NORPACE	RYTHMODAN
dobutamine	DOBUTREX	
dopamine	INTROPIN	
epinephrine	EPIPEN, PRIMATENE MIST, TWINJECT, ADRENALIN, ADRENACLICK	EPIPEN
esmolol	BREVIBLOC, ESMOLOL HCL	BREVIBLOC
flecainide	TAMBOCOR	
gemfibrozil	LOPID	
guanethidine	ISMELIN	
hydralazine	APRESOLINE	
ibutilide	CORVERT	
labetalol	NORMODYNE, TRANDATE	TRANDATE
lidocaine	LIDODERM, XYLOCAINE, TOPICAINE, ZILACTIN-L, BURNAMYCIN	XYLOCAINE
lovastatin	ALTOPREV, MEVACOR	MEVACOR, ADVICOR
mecamylamine	INVERSINE	
methyldopa	ALDOMET	METHYLDOPA
metoprolol	TOPROL	BETALOC, LOPRESSOR
metyrosine	DEMSER	
mexiletine	MEXITIL	MEXILITINE
milrinone	PRIMACOR	MILRINONE INJECTION

DRUGS IN THIS CHAPTER (continued)

Generic Name	US Trade Name	Canadian Trade Name
minoxidil	LONITEN, ROGAINE	
niacin	NIASPAN, SIO-NIACIN, NIACOR, NIACINOL, NICOTINEX	NIACIN, ADVICOR
nifedipine	ADALAT, PROCARDIA, AFEDITAB, NIFEDIAC, NIFEDICAL	ADALAT
nitroglycerin	MINITRAN, NITRO (-BID, -DUR, LINGUAL, STAT, TAB, MIST), NITREK	MINITRAN, NITRATES, NITRO (-DUR, LINGUAL, STAT), NITROL
norepinephrine	LEVOPHED	
orlistat	XENICAL, ALLI	XENICAL
phentolamine	REGITINE, ORAVERSE	ROGITINE
phenylephrine	AK-DILATE, NEOFRIN, NOSTRIL, PREFRIN, OCU-PHRIN, VICKS SINEX, MYDFRIN	AK-DILATE, AK-VERNACON, BENYLIN, CLEAR EYES, CONTAC, DAYQUIL, DIMETAPP
prazosin	MINIPRESS	
procainamide	PROCANBID, PRONESTYL	PROCAN-SR

Generic Name	US Trade Name	Canadian Trade Name
propafenone	RYTHMOL	
propranolol	INDERAL, AVLOCARDYL, DERALIN, DOCITON, INDERALICI, BEDRANOL SR	INDERAL-LA
pseudoephedrine	SUDAFED, DIMETAPP DECONGESTANT, SIMPLY STUFFY, CENAFED, CONTAC 12-HOUR, BIOFED	SUDAFED, DIMETAPP DECONGESTANT, CONTAC COLD-NASAL CONGESTION
quinidine	QUINAGLUTE, QUINALAN	QUINIDINE
reserpine	RESA, SERPALAN	
sodium nitroprusside	NITROPRESS	NIPRIDE
sotalol	BETAPACE, SORINE	
timolol	TIMOPTIC, OCUDOSE, BLOCADREN, ISTALOL	TIMOPTIC
tocainide	TONOCARD	
vasopressin	PITRESSIN	PRESSYN
verapamil	CALAN, COVERA-HS, ISOPTIN, VERELAN	COVERA-HS

Cardiac Electrophysiology

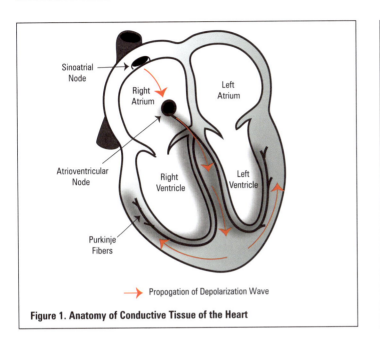

Figure 1. Anatomy of Conductive Tissue of the Heart

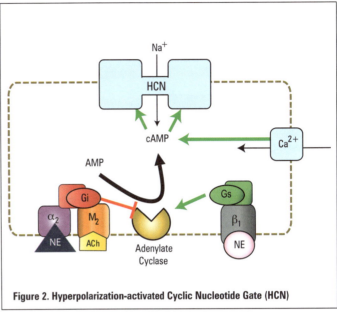

Figure 2. Hyperpolarization-activated Cyclic Nucleotide Gate (HCN)

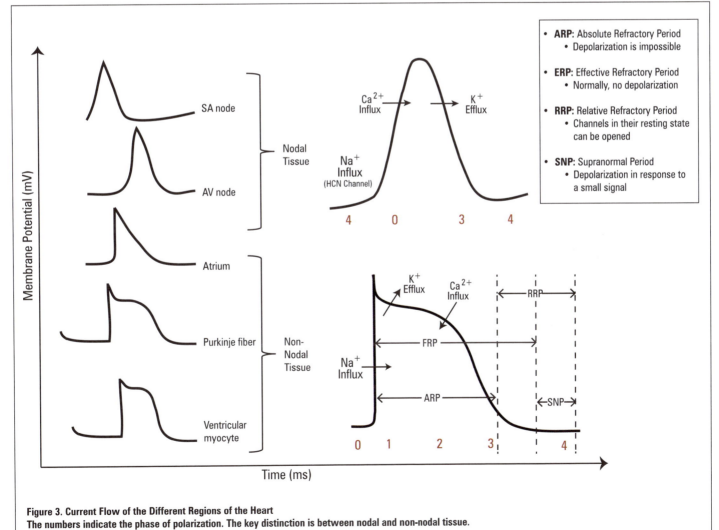

- **ARP:** Absolute Refractory Period
  - Depolarization is impossible
- **ERP:** Effective Refractory Period
  - Normally, no depolarization
- **RRP:** Relative Refractory Period
  - Channels in their resting state can be opened
- **SNP:** Supranormal Period
  - Depolarization in response to a small signal

Figure 3. Current Flow of the Different Regions of the Heart
The numbers indicate the phase of polarization. The key distinction is between nodal and non-nodal tissue.

Antiarrhythmics

Three Mechanisms of Arrhythmia

Arrhythmia occurs when the normal sequence of impulse initiation and propagation is altered through three mechanisms.

Abnormal Automaticity
- Increased or decreased SA node pacing

Triggered Activity
- Injured cardiac myocytes undergo premature depolarization generating ectopic beats

Re-entry
- Backward conduction along an abnormal portion of the heart circuitry
  - Most clinically important arrhythmias (atrial fibrillation, atrial flutter, AV-node re-entry tachycardia (e.g. Wolff-Parkinson-White), post-MI ventricular tachycardia, and ventricular fibrillation)

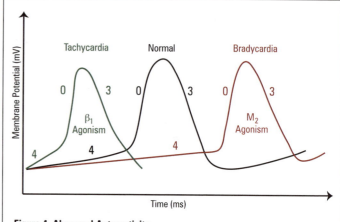

Figure 4. Abnormal Automaticity

Four Classes of Antiarrhythmics

I. Na+ channel blockers (also local anesthetics)
   Class Ia: QUINIDINE, AMIODARONE, PROCAINAMIDE, DISOPYRAMIDE

   Class Ib: LIDOCAINE, MEXILETINE, TOCAINIDE

   Class Ic: FLECAINIDE, ENCAINIDE, PROPAFENONE

II. β Blockers
    PROPANOLOL, ESMOLOL, METOPROLOL, ATENOLOL, TIMOLOL

III. K+ channel blockers
     SOTALOL, IBUTILIDE, BRETYLIUM, AMIODARONE (class Ia & III)

IV. Ca2+ channel blockers
    VERAPAMIL, DILTIAZEM

Others: ADENOSINE, ATROPINE, DIGOXIN (see Cardiac Inotropes)

Effect of Antiarrhythmics on Conductive Tissue of the Heart

SA Node
- **Class I drugs** slow phase 4 depolarization
- **Class II drugs** slow phase 0 depolarization
- **Class IV drugs** slow phase 0 depolarization

AV Node
- **Class I drugs** slow phase 4 depolarization
- **Class II drugs** block β1-receptor, decrease cAMP, decrease Na+ influx, slow phase 4 depolarization
- **Class IV drugs** inhibit phase 0 directly, inhibit phase 4 indirectly
- **Others:** ADENOSINE and DIGOXIN

Atrium
- **Class I drugs** slow phase 0 but have different effects on phase 3 (depending on class subtype)
- **Class III drugs** slow phase 3

Purkinje/Ventricle
- **Class I drugs** slow phase 0 but have different effects on phase 3 (depending on class subtype)
- **Class II drugs** block β1-receptor found throughout the ventricle (AV node is more sensitive)
- **Class III drugs** slow phase 3

All antiarrhythmics can cause arrhythmia

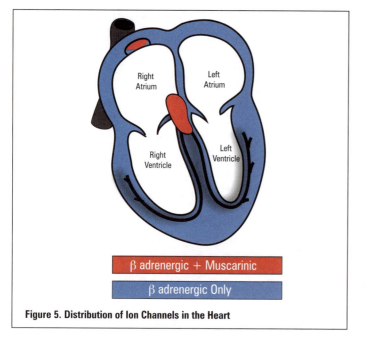

Figure 5. Distribution of Ion Channels in the Heart

Antiarrhythmics

Class IA Drugs

Drug	QUINIDINE	PROCAINAMIDE	DISOPYRAMIDE
MOA	• Blocks Na+ channels, with some K+ channel block • Nodal tissue: slows phase 4 depolarization • Non-nodal tissue: slows rate of phase 0 rise • Slows conduction (negative inotropy) • Prolongs action potential and ERP • QT prolongation	• Blocks Na+ channels, with some K+ channel block • Nodal tissue: slows phase 4 depolarization • Non-nodal tissue: slows rate of phase 0 rise • Slows conduction (negative inotropy) • Prolongs action potential and ERP	• Blocks Na+ channels, with some K+ channel block • Nodal tissue: slows phase 4 depolarization • Non-nodal tissue: slows rate of phase 0 rise • Slows conduction (negative inotropy) • Prolongs action potential and ERP
USES	• Atrial and ventricular arrhythmias (flutter, fibrillation) • NOT effective for arrhythmias originating in the nodes • Malaria	• Atrial and ventricular arrhythmias (flutter, fibrillation) • NOT effective for arrhythmias originating in the nodes	• Atrial and ventricular arrhythmias (flutter, fibrillation) • NOT effective for arrhythmias originating in the nodes
PK	• Moderate $t_{1/2}$ (6-8 hours) • Hepatic metabolism (appropriate for patients with renal failure)	• Short $t_{1/2}$ (2-4 hours) • Dose adjustment needed in renal failure	• Moderate $t_{1/2}$ (6-9 hours) • Mixed hepatic metabolism and renal excretion – dose adjustment needed in renal failure
ADRs	• Torsades de pointes (especially patients with long QT syndrome) • Diarrhea • Thrombocytopenia • Antimuscarinic effects (BLUSHPADS BBC) • Vasodilation (hypotension) • Cinchonism = headache + tinnitus (dizziness, hearing loss)	• Diarrhea • Thrombocytopenia • Antimuscarinic effects (BLUSHPADS BBC) • Vasodilation (hypotension) • Reversible lupus-like syndrome	• Diarrhea • Thrombocytopenia • Antimuscarinic effects (BLUSHPADS BBC) • Vasodilation (hypotension)
CONTRAINDICATIONS	• Complete AV block • Myasthenia gravis	• Complete AV block • Systemic lupus erythematosus (SLE)	• Complete AV block
INTERACTIONS	• Can displace DIGOXIN from tissue sites and decrease its renal elimination leading to an increase in DIGOXIN serum levels by up to 100%		

Class IB Drugs

Drug	LIDOCAINE	MEXILETINE	TOCAINIDE
MOA	• Shortens action potential – greater effect in partially depolarized cells such as diseased Purkinje and ventricular tissue • Slight slowing of conduction		
USES	• Ventricular arrhythmias (in patient – post MI to prevent ventricular tachycardia and/or ventricular fibrillation) • NOT useful for treating arrhythmias originating in the atria • Digitalis-induced arrhythmias		
PK	• Extensive first pass metabolism – given IV only • Short $t_{1/2}$ (100 minutes) • Hepatic metabolism	• High bioavailability – oral administration • Moderate $t_{1/2}$ (9-12 hours) • Hepatic metabolism	• High bioavailability – oral administration • Long $t_{1/2}$ (11-15 hours) • Lower hepatic metabolism than LIDOCAINE/MEXILETINE
ADRs	• CNS stimulation or depression (paresthesia, drowsiness) • Bradycardia, lightheadedness • Convulsions with toxic doses • Anorexia, nausea		
CONTRAINDICATIONS	• Cardiogenic shock • AV Block		
NOTES	• This is the LEAST toxic class of antiarrhythmic drugs – minimal ECG effects		

Antiarrhythmics

Class IC Drugs

Drug	FLECAINIDE	PROPAFENONE
MOA	• Slows maximum rate of depolarization • Slowing of conduction • QT, QRS and PR prolongation	
USES	• Last-resort treatment of atrial or ventricular tachycardia, which can progress to ventricular fibrillation if untreated • Treatment of intractable SVT	
PK	• Long $t_{1/2}$ (16-20 hours) • Hepatic metabolism	• Clearance is dose dependant – higher dose has lower clearance • Almost completely metabolized by the liver
ADRs	• Arrhythmia • Dizziness, blurred vision	
CONTRAINDICATIONS	• Contraindicated post-MI (due to pro-arrhythmogenicity)	
NOTES	• No effect of Class Ic on action potential duration	

Class II Drugs – β-Blockers

Drug	PROPRANOLOL, ESMOLOL, METOPROLOL, ATENOLOL, TIMOLOL
MOA	• Prolongs phases 4 and 0 in SA and AV nodes • Antagonism of β-receptors decreases intracellular cAMP → decreased "funny" and Ca^{2+} currents in nodal cells • Result is longer PR interval
USES	• Arrhythmias arising either in the atria or the ventricles • Tachycardias due to sympathetic stimulation or post-anesthesia • AV nodal re-entry supraventricular tachy (atrial fibrillation or flutter) • Stops AV conductance
PK, ADRs, CONTRAINDICATIONS	• Please see β-blocker section

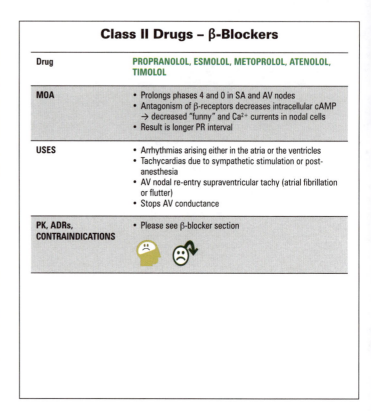

Class III Drugs

Drug	BRETYLIUM	AMIODARONE	SOTALOL
MOA	• Block K^+ channels in all regions of the heart • Prolongs action potential duration and ERP		
USES	• Prophylaxis of ventricular tachycardia and ventricular fibrillation (outpatient) • Treatment of atrial flutter and atrial fibrillation		
PK	• Moderate $t_{1/2}$ (6-10 hours) • Mostly renal excretion	• Very long $t_{1/2}$ (20-50 days) • Hepatic metabolism	• Long $t_{1/2}$ (13 hours) • Renal excretion (100%)

ADRs	• Arrhythmia
	• Cardiovascular block
	• Bradycardia
	• CHF
		• Arrhythmia
		• Cardiovascular block
		• Bradycardia
		• CHF
		• Contains iodine, which can lead to:
		  • Pulmonary fibrosis
		  • Hepatotoxicity
		  • Thyroid dysfunction
		  • Corneal deposits
		  • Photodermatitus
		  • Neurologic problems
		  • Constipation
			• Arrhythmia
			• Cardiovascular block
			• Bradycardia
			• CHF

CONTRAINDICATIONS	• Cardiogenic shock • Marked sinus bradycardia		
NOTES	• IBUTILIDE and DOFETILID are also Class III antiarrhythmics with a very low therapeutic index and thus are only used in the hospital setting		

Antiarrhythmics

Class IV Drugs – Ca²⁺ Channel Blockers

Drug	Calcium Channel Blockers – **VERAPAMIL, DILTIAZEM**
MOA	• Prolong phase 0 in SA and AV nodes to slow conduction • Prolongs ERP and the PR interval
USES	• Prevention of nodal arrhythmias (supraventricular or tachycardia) • Prevent spread of arrhythmia to ventricle • NOT useful for an arrhythmia originating in the ventricle (e.g. variant (Prinzmetal's) angina)
PK	• See Vasodilators section
ADRs	• See Vasodilators section
CONTRAINDICATIONS	• See Vasodilators section
NOTES	• Dihydropyridine-type Ca²⁺ channel blockers are NOT useful antiarrhythmics, as these drugs are more selective for vasculature and may precipitate reflex tachycardia

Other

Drug	**ADENOSINE**

MOA	• Binds to adenosine (A_1) receptor, leading to:
	  • Decreased cAMP formation and a longer phase 4
	  • Decreased Ca²⁺ channel opening in response to norepinephrine, leading to a longer phase 0
	• Slows conduction through AV node

USES	• Diagnosis and treatment of acute AV nodal arrhythmias (very short-acting) • Tachycardia • Multifocal atrial tachycardia and AV nodal reentry supraventricular tachycardia (drug acts to stop AV conductance of atrial fibrillation and atrial flutter)
PK	• Very short $t_{1/2}$ (seconds)
ADRs	• Flushing • Bronchoconstriction (avoid in patients with asthma or COPD) • Ventricular fibrillation/flutter may result from concurrent administration of adenosine with **DIGOXIN** or **DIGOXIN** and **VERAPAMIL** in combination
CONTRAINDICATIONS	• Heart transplant patients (very sensitive to effects of **ADENOSINE**)
NOTES	• **ADENOSINE** is a normal metabolite of ATP, indicating high energy usage. During periods of high energy usage, **ADENOSINE** causes vasodilation in order to increase blood flow

Why can antiarrhythmic drugs cause arrhythmia?

- Prolonging action potential (AP) duration and ARP can cause an early after-depolarization either if an arrhythmia is borderline (slightly prolonged AP) or in the case of delayed after-depolarization
- This mechanism of iatrogenic arrhythmia is due to AP prolongation and therefore can be caused by **AMIODARONE** or **QUINIDINE**, among other drugs
- AP prolongation can also result in Torsades de Pointes
- Blocking aberrant conduction through the Purkinje system aims to block backward current while preserving forward current. Treatment may, however, block forward current while allowing some backward current to persist, precipitating arrhythmia

Shock

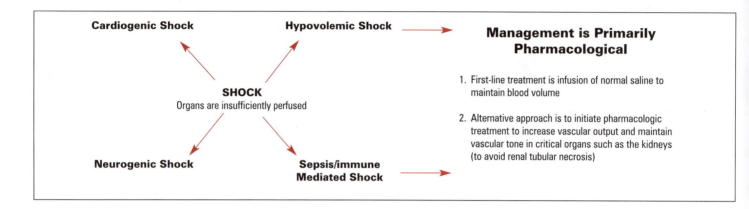

Management is Primarily Pharmacological

1. First-line treatment is infusion of normal saline to maintain blood volume

2. Alternative approach is to initiate pharmacologic treatment to increase vascular output and maintain vascular tone in critical organs such as the kidneys (to avoid renal tubular necrosis)

Neurogenic Shock

- Caused by head trauma which increases parasympathetic outflow, thereby counteracting the sympathetic tone required for normal cardiovascular function
- Management includes:
  - Supportive therapy - brain will eventually "reboot," restoring vascular tone and cardiac output
  - **NOREPINEPHRINE** if hemorrhage has been ruled out

Cardiogenic Shock

- Common causes:
  - Acute or chronic LV dysfunction
  - Myocardial rupture or acute ventricular septal defect following MI
  - Acute valvular regurgitation
  - β-blocker or Ca^{2+} channel blocker overdose
- Often occurs with pulmonary edema

Sepsis/Immune Mediated Shock

- Massive cytokine release causes massive vasodilation

Hypovolemic Shock

- Insufficient blood volume, commonly caused by:
  - Dehydration
  - Trauma
  - Small, slow bleeding

Drugs Used in the Treatment of Shock

EPINEPHRINE
MOA
- Agonizes β_1-receptors to ↑ HR and maintain perfusion (MOST IMPORTANT MOA)
- Agonizes β_2-receptors to maintain renal and muscular perfusion and to maintain air flow in the lungs
- Agonizes α_1-receptors to maintain vascular tone

DOBUTAMINE
- See Positive Inotrope section

DOPAMINE
MOA
- Effects are dose-dependent
  - Highest dose:
    - Acts as an α_1-agonist to induce vasoconstriction
  - Medium dose:
    - Acts as a β_1-agonist to increase heart inotropy and HR
  - Lowest dose:
    - Binds to D_1-receptors on vascular smooth muscle cells of the abdominal viscera to cause selective dilation of renal and splanchnic blood vessels, thereby preventing loss of blood supply to these organs
    - Binds to presynaptic D_2-receptors to reduce α-adrenergic stimulation on smooth muscle – increases renal blood flow

VASOPRESSIN
- See Diuretics section

Vasodilators and Vasoconstrictors

Autonomic nervous system malfunctions are important contributors to elevations of systemic vasomotor tone. This produces vasoconstriction resulting in increased peripheral vascular resistance and consequent systemic arterial hypertension. Systemic arterial hypertension is a known positive antecedent event correlated with cardiac hypertrophy, heart failure and stroke.

- The principal sites of action for drugs which modulate the autonomic nervous system to lower blood pressure include:

  1. Autonomic ganglia
  2. Autonomic nerve termini
  3. Sympathetic receptors
     - β_1-adrenoceptors
     - Heart (cardiac rate and contractility)
     - Juxtaglomerular complex in the kidney – renin release (and, consequently, angiotensin and aldosterone production)
     - α_1-adrenoceptors on vascular smooth muscle cells of blood vessels which mediate vasoconstriction

Adrenergic Receptor Actions in the Human Cardiovascular System

Epinephrine is a non-selective adrenergic agonist
- Physiologic levels of epinephrine primarily agonize β_1- and β_2-receptors
- Pharmacologic doses of epinephrine are higher and primarily agonize α_1 because of the relative excess of α-receptors compared with β-receptors

Receptor Distribution
- α_2-agonists generally result in vasodilation by release of nitric oxide, a smooth muscle relaxant
- β_1- and β_2-agonists generally result in vasodilation by smooth muscle relaxation (recall, β_1-adrenoceptors generally found in the heart and coronary blood vessels; β_2-adrenoceptors found in the periphery, e.g. lungs)

Antihypertensives

Many drug classes can produce antihypertensive effects, including:
- Diuretics
- Sympatholytics
- Ca^{2+} channel blockers
- ACE inhibitors
- Angiotensin II-receptor antagonists (ARBs)
- Vasodilators

Vasoconstrictors

PHENYLEPHRINE

MOA
- α_1-adrenoceptor agonists acting on peripheral vasculature
- α_1-agonists generally result in vasoconstriction by smooth muscle contraction, with minimal effect on β-adrenoceptors (unless at high doses)

USES
- Decongestant – vasoconstriction resulting from intranasal application
- Pressor agent – elevate blood pressure by increasing peripheral resistance, especially in hypotensive patients on spinal anesthesia
- Anti-allergy

PK
- Short $t_{1/2}$ (2-3 hours)

ADRs
- Hypertension
- Rebound nasal congestion
- Eye pain

CONTRAINDICATIONS
- Breastfeeding mothers/newborns
- Severe hypertension
- Closed angle glaucoma

NOTES
- Desensitization may occur
- Other examples include: **PSEUDOEPHEDRINE**

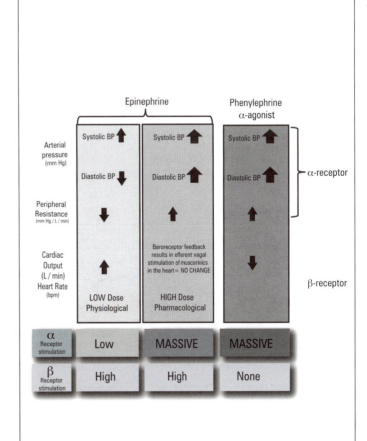

Figure 6. Effects of α- and β-receptor Stimulation on Systemic Blood Flow

Nitrovasodilators

MOA
- Two major mechanisms
  1. Venous dilation (decreases preload, thereby decreasing oxygen demand)
  2. Arteriolar/coronary vasodilation (NO is formed, which both activates guanylyl cyclase to increase cGMP and directly stimulates K^+ channels; the end result of either mechanism is to relax venous vasculature)
     - While endogenous NO is formed in endothelial cells, exogenous nitrates form NO in an endothelial cell-independent manner

USES
- Acute angina due to chronic, stable angina (decreases oxygen demand)
- Acute angina due to variant (Prinzmetal's) angina (halts vasospasm)
- Acute angina due to unstable angina (decreased oxygen demand AND decreased vasospasm)
  - NOT useful for continuous therapy, due to rapid development of tolerance
  - Used as intermittant prescription to prevent tolerance
- Other uses: treatment of pulmonary edema

PK
- Very low oral bioavailability due to liver metabolism (Isosorbide mononitrate is an exception)
- Sublingual administration bypasses the oral route

ADRs
- Due to blood pooling in veins and not returning to heart
- Headache
- Postural hypotension
- Reflex tachycardia
- Rapid tolerance
- Paradoxical angina (if coronary atherosclerosis is proximal in the artery)

CONTRAINDICATIONS
- **SILDENAFIL** (may cause CV collapse and massive shock)
- Elevated intracranial pressure

AMYL NITRITE
PK
- Onset very rapid (seconds to minutes)

ADRs
- Cardiovascular toxicity due to abuse by inhalation

NITROGLYCERIN
USES
- Commonly used as a vasodilator/anti-anginal in the clinical setting

PK
- Very short $t_{1/2}$ (3 minutes)
- Sublingual administration is preferred to avoid first-pass metabolism

ADRs
- Tolerance, may develop very quickly

SODIUM NITROPRUSSIDE
USES
- Used to treat an acute, hypertensive crisis
- Congestive heart failure

PK
- Very short $t_{1/2}$ (2 minutes)

ADRs
- Rebound hypertension upon withdrawal
- Cyanide and thiocyanate toxicity (by-products of drug metabolism)
- Uncouple ETC to cause respiratory failure and lactic acid accumulation due to muscle failure
- May cause eventual ataxia and optic neuropathy

CONTRAINDICATIONS
- Patients with hypovolemia
- Congestive heart failure with reduced peripheral vascular resistance
- Patients with optic atrophy or tobacco amblyopia

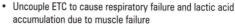

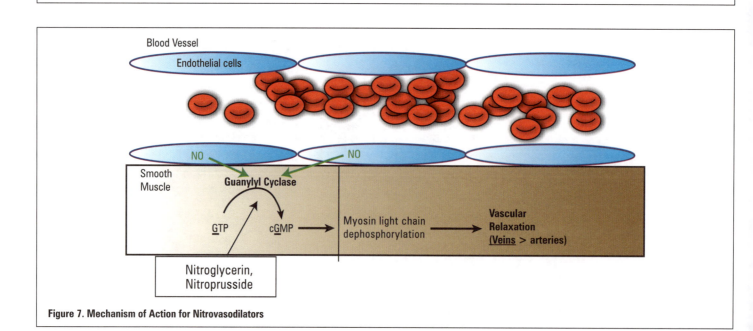

Figure 7. Mechanism of Action for Nitrovasodilators

Sympatholytic/Anti-Adrenergic Drugs

METYROSINE
MOA
- Blocks catecholamine synthesis by inhibiting tyrosine hydroxylase

USES
- Treatment of pheochromocytoma symptoms

PK
- Short $t_{1/2}$ (3-4 hours)

ADRs
- Extrapyramidal signs due to reduced dopaminergic transmission
- Impotence
- Diarrhea
- Sedation
- Galactorrhea
- Dysuria

CONTRAINDICATIONS
- Hypersensitivity to METYROSINE products

NOTES
- Crosses the BBB

GUANETHIDINE
MOA
- Two phases:
  1. Depletes NE stores via rapid firing
  2. Prevents NE release

USES
- Moderate hypertension

PK
- Very long $t_{1/2}$ (5-10 days)

ADRs
- Na+/water retention → higher BP, edema
- Sexual dysfunction
- Orthostatic hypotension

CONTRAINDICATIONS
- Pheochromocytoma (rapid release of NE from pheo)
- MAOI therapy
- Heart failure

RESERPINE
MOA
- Depletes central and peripheral stores of vesicular NE by blocking catecholamine uptake into vesicles

USES
- Used for the treatment of mild hypertension
- Psychotic disorder

PK
- Very long $t_{1/2}$ (8-9 days)

ADRs
- Depression
- Sedation
- Extrapyramidal signs
- Cardiac dysrhythmia
- Gastrointestinal hemorrhage

CONTRAINDICATIONS
- Active depression
- Active peptic ulcer disease
- Active gastrointestinal disease
- Severe renal failure
- Ulcerative colitis

MECAMYLAMINE
MOA
- Nicotinic acetylcholine receptor antagonist – blocks stimulation of post-ganglionic nerve

USES
- Severe or malignant hypertension

PK
- Long $t_{1/2}$ (24 hours)

ADRs (due to ganglionic block)
- Orthostatic hypotension and syncope
- Paralytic ileus
- Dizziness, sedation and fatigue

CONTRAINDICATIONS
- Coronary insufficiency
- Glaucoma
- Myocardial infarction (recent)
- Patients on antibiotics or sulfonamides
- Pyloric stenosis
- Renal insufficiency and/or uremia

NOTES
- Ganglionic blockers affect both sympathetic and parasympathetic ganglia and the side effects are dependent on the dominant tone in the organ system
- Other examples include: HEXAMETHONIUM, PENTOLINIUM

CLONIDINE
MOA
- Two phases of action:
  1. Initial phase is peripheral: stimulates α_1-receptors, causing transient vasoconstriction
  2. Second phase is central: binding to CNS α_2-receptors diminishes all noradrenergic outflow and reduces blood pressure via decreased total peripheral resistance, decreased HR, and decreased renin release

USES
- Hypertension
- Tobacco/opioid withdrawal (prevents reflex vasoconstriction)
- Intrathecal analgesia

PK
- Long $t_{1/2}$ (12-16 hours)
- Renal excretion

ADRs
- Rebound hypertension if discontinued abruptly
- Dry mouth
- Sedation
- Hypotension (particularly with epidural administration)

CONTRAINDICATIONS
- Anticoagulant therapy
- Bleeding diathesis
- Epidural administration above C4 dermatome

METHYLDOPA
MOA
- Converted to α-methyl-norepinephrine (a potent α_2-agonist)

USES
- Hypertension

PK
- Short $t_{1/2}$ (2 hours)

ADRs
- Lethargy
- Depression
- Hemolytic anemia
- Impotence

CONTRAINDICATIONS
- Liver disease
- MAOI therapy

α-Blockers

PHENTOLAMINE
MOA
- Blocks α_1- and α_2-receptors

USES
- Hypertension (e.g. secondary to pheochromocytoma)
- Treatment for norepinephrine adverse reaction

PK
- Short $t_{1/2}$ (2-3 hours)

ADRs
- Major side effect is orthostatic hypotension
- Diarrhea
- Nasal congestion
- Cardiac dysrhythmia

CONTRAINDICATIONS
- Angina
- Coronary artery disease
- Recent myocardial infarction

PRAZOSIN
MOA
- Blocks α_1-receptors selectively
- Preferred over nonselective α blockers

USES
- Hypertension

PK
- Short $t_{1/2}$ (2-3 hours)

ADRs
- Orthostatic hypotension
- Nausea

CONTRAINDICATIONS
- Precautions with concomitant use of other antihypertensives, β-blockers, diuretics

Sympatholytic/Anti-Adrenergic Drugs

Common Features of all β-blockers

COMMON ADRs
- Cardiac depression
- Sexual dysfunction
- No tachycardia in response to diabetic hypoglycemia
- Fatigue
- Cold extremities
- Bradycardia

COMMON CONTRAINDICATIONS
- Asthma (particularly with non-selective β-blockers)
- 2nd or 3rd degree conduction block
- Stage 4 CHF or CHF with hypotension

Peripheral Effects of β-Blockers

- Decrease cardiac output
- Decrease renin release
- Useful in the treatment of hypertension

(see *Negative Inotropes* for more information on cardiac effects of β-blockers)

PROPRANOLOL
MOA
- Blocks β_1- and β_2-receptors

METOPROLOL
MOA
- β_1-receptor blocker

Mixed Blockers

CARVEDILOL and **LABETALOL**
MOA
- Blocks α_1-, β_1- and β_2-receptors

USES
- Treat stage 2 and 3 congestive heart failure

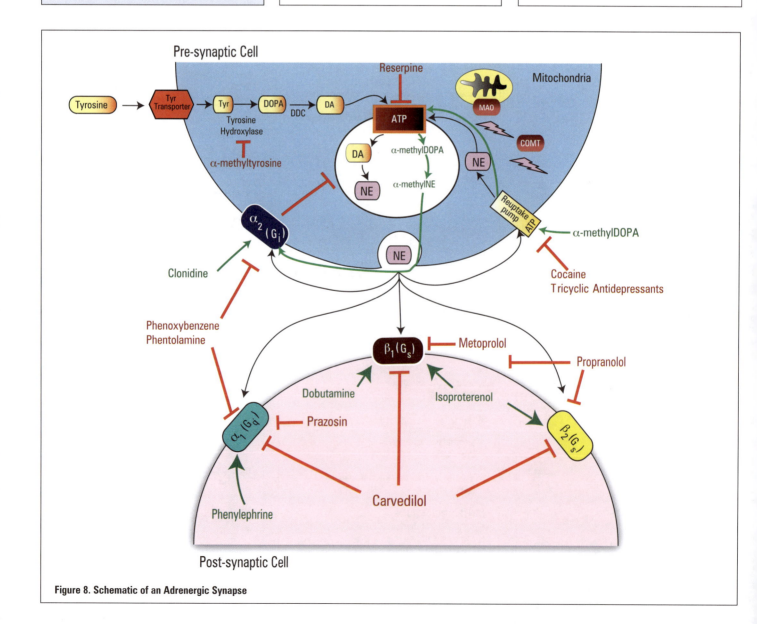

Figure 8. Schematic of an Adrenergic Synapse

Non-Autonomic Vasodilators

- Activate renin-angiotensin-aldosterone axis that will cause sodium and water reabsorption and potassium loss
- Tachycardia = not good for heart failure

HYDRALAZINE
MOA
- Increases cGMP to elicit smooth muscle relaxation
  - Vasodilates arterioles more than veins (reduces afterload)

USES
- First-line treatment for treatment of hypertension in pregnancy
- Severe hypertension
- Congestive heart failure

ADRs
- Lupus-like syndrome, including a facial malar rash
- Hepatotoxicity
- Leukopenia
- Tachycardia
- Headache
- GI distress

CONTRAINDICATIONS
- Dissecting aortic aneurysm
- Liver disease
- Coronary or cerebrovascular disease

Potassium Channel Activators

DIAZOXIDE
MOA
- Activation of K^+-ATPase channels in vascular smooth muscle, resulting in vasodilation
- Inhibits insulin secretion from pancreatic β-cells

USES
- Malignant hypertension (e.g. pre-eclampsia during pregnancy)
- Hypertensive emergencies
- Hypoglycemia due to hyperinsulinism

PK
- Very long $t_{1/2}$ (21-36 hours)

ADRs
- Hirsutism
- Hyperglycemia
- Hypotension
- Reflex tachycardia
- Uterine relaxation

CONTRAINDICATIONS
- Pheochromocytoma
- Functional hypoglycemia

MINOXIDIL
MOA
- Opens potassium channels

USES
- Severe, refractory hypertension
- Topical stimulation of hair growth

PK
- Moderate $t_{1/2}$ (4-5 hours)

ADRs
- Can cause pericardial effusion progressing to tamponade
- Hypotension
- Hirsutism
- Hypernatremia, fluid retention
- Tachycardia

CONTRAINDICATIONS
- Pheochromocytoma
- Coronary or cerebrovascular disease

Non-autonomic Vasodilators

Calcium Channel-Blocking Drugs

- There are 3 types of calcium channel blockers and they differ in their relative selectivity toward cardiac vs. vascular L-type calcium channels
  - Phenylalkylamines are coronary dilators (e.g. **VERAPAMIL**)
  - Benzothiazepines are coronary and peripheral dilators (e.g. **DILTIAZEM**)
  - Dihydropyridines are peripheral dilators (e.g. **NIFEDIPINE**)

MOA
- Calcium channel blockers bind to the L-type calcium channel, blocking calcium flow into the myocyte, and resulting in:
  - **Arterial dilation**
    - **NIFEDIPINE > DILTIAZEM > VERAPAMIL**
  - Depressed myocardial **contraction, conduction** and **pacemaker** rate
    - **VERAPAMIL > DILTIAZEM > NIFEDIPINE**
  - Intrinsic natriuretic diuretic effect

ADRs
- Mainly due to vasodilation
  - Flushing
  - Headache
  - Edema

Coronary Dilators

VERAPAMIL

MOA
- Unselective Ca^{2+} channel binding in both the heart and vascular smooth muscle results in:
  - Decreased arterial pressure
  - Decreased cardiac contractility (opposes baroreceptor-mediated tachycardia)
  - Slowed SA and AV nodal conduction

USES
- Hypertension
- Monotherapy for the treatment of angina (causes coronary vasodilation in addition to peripheral vasodilation)
- Management of supraventricular arrhythmias

PK
- Moderate $t_{1/2}$ (5-12 hours)

ADRs
- Cardiac depression
- Constipation (unique, due to reduced gut motility)

CONTRAINDICATIONS
- Patients with heart damage (cardiodepression exacerbates impairment of pacing and conduction)
- Patients taking β-blockers (slows nodes)

NOTES
- Phenylalkylamines class

Coronary and Peripheral Dilators

DILTIAZEM

MOA
- Targets mainly vascular smooth muscle to decrease arterial pressure

USES
- Angina monotherapy
- Hypertension
- Paroxysmal supraventricular tachycardia (atrial flutter and/or fibrillation)

PK
- Short $t_{1/2}$ (3-5 hours)

ADRs
- **Mild** cardiodepression (less than **VERAPAMIL**)
- Unlike **VERAPAMIL**, does NOT cause constipation

CONTRAINDICATIONS
- Contraindicated in patients with heart disease because of cardiodepression

NOTES
- Benzothiazepine class
- Unlike other calcium channel blockers, can be used in conjunction with a β-blocker

Peripheral Dilators

AMLODIPINE

MOA
- Binding to Ca^{2+} channels is selective for vascular smooth muscle
- Results in greater decrease in blood pressure than **DILTIAZEM** or **VERAPAMIL** with no cardiodepression

USES
- Peripheral hypertension

PK
- Very long $t_{1/2}$ (30-50 hours)

ADRs
- Not as well tolerated as **DILTIAZEM** and **VERAPAMIL**
- Peripheral edema that does not respond to diuretics.
- Reflex tachycardia (due to lack of cardiodepression) that may worsen angina or cause cardiac palpitations
- Long half-life means slow onset of therapeutic effects and side effects

CONTRAINDICATIONS
- Ischemic heart disease (angina, MI)
- Pregnancy – limb bud defects
- Prolonged labour (relaxed uterine smooth muscle)

NOTES
- Dihydropyridine class
- Other example of this class include: **NIFEDIPINE**

Heart Failure: Introduction

Congestive Heart Failure Overview

Definition
- Congestive heart failure is the inability of the heart to maintain a cardiac output necessary to meet metabolic demands and the venous return

Classification - General
- "Backward" Heart Failure: heart can only accept venous return at high filling pressures, resulting in (left heart dysfunction) pulmonary congestion or (right-heart dysfunction) peripheral edema
- "Forward" Heart Failure: left-heart is unable to eject blood at sufficient rate to meet metabolic demands of body
- Compensatory mechanisms try to maintain cardiac output and blood pressure
  - Frank-Starling mechanism
  - Sympathetic nervous system (increased heart rate, increased contractility)
  - Myocardial hypertrophy
  - Fluid retention (renal effect)

New York Heart Association Classification of Heart Failure

Class I	Patient has cardiovascular disease, but no symptoms with ordinary physical activity (i.e. climbing stairs)
Class II	Symptoms with ordinary physical activity resulting in mild limitations, but no symptoms at rest
Class III	Symptoms with less than normal physical activity resulting in severe limitations, patients are only comfortable at rest
Class IV	Symptoms with any physical activity, symptoms may even be present at rest

Risk Factors
- Predisposing conditions of heart failure:
  1. Coronary heart disease with infarction
  2. Hypertension
  3. Non-ischemic cardiomyopathy
  4. Diabetes
  5. Valvular heart disease
- Heart failure occurs due to:
  1. Impaired contractility
  2. Increased afterload
  3. Impaired ventricular filling
- Cellular and molecular causes:
  - Abnormal energy metabolism
  - Cytoskeletal abnormalities
  - Altered contractile proteins
  - Altered β-adrenergics
  - Abnormal myocyte excitation/contraction coupling

The following drugs are contraindicated in heart failure:
- Positive inotropes (except in Stage D)
- Certain antiarrhythmics (except Class II agents)
- Ca^{2+} channel blockers (**DILTIAZEM** and **VERAPAMIL**) and negative inotropes
- NSAIDs
- High dose cardiac glycosides (except in Stage D)

Currently there is evidence that the following drugs decrease mortality in heart failure:
- β-blockers
- ACE inhibitors/angiotensin receptor blockers (ARBs)
- Spironolactone

Vasodilators Worsen Heart Failure

If a vasodilator is used chronically in a patient with heart failure, the blood vessels develop decreased tone and larger capacitance. The larger capacitance will allow for a greater blood volume, but the failing heart still will not be able to move blood. Recall, HF is not an afterload/vascular tension problem, it is a failure of the heart to move blood.

The first line drug for controlling hypertension in a patient with HF is an ACE inhibitor or angiotensin receptor blocker, NOT a vasodilator or diuretic. Diuretics are used for pulmonary congestion and not hypertension.

Heart Failure

STAGE A (1)
Defining characteristics
- High risk of developing heart failure, but no structural abnormalities and no symptoms

Typical patient has...
- The predisposing conditions listed on left

Overview of therapeutic approach
- Tailor treatment to the patient's predisposing conditions (i.e diuretics for hypertension), but always include dietary and lifestyle changes

STAGE B (2)
Defining characteristics
- Structural heart disease, but no symptoms

Typical patient has...
- Previous MI, LVH, low LVEF, and/or asymptomatic valvular disease

Overview of therapeutic approach
- Same as above plus ACE inhibitors/angiotensin receptor blockers and/or β-blockers in appropriate patients
  - ACE inhibitors → lower BP
  - β-blockers → lower HR and BP

STAGE C (3)
Defining characteristics
- Structural heart disease with current or prior symptoms

Typical patient has...
- Now developed symptoms

Overview of therapeutic approach
Same as above but
- Routine drugs: diuretics, ACE inhibitors, **β-blockers**
- Selected drugs: aldosterone antagonist, ARB, **DIGITALIS**, **HYDRALAZINE**
- Selected devices: biventricular pacers and/or defibrillators

STAGE D (4)
Defining characteristics
- Refractory heart failure (Class IV) requiring specialized intervention

Typical patient has...
- Symptoms despite maximal medical therapy with serial hospitalizations

Overview of therapeutic approach
Same as above but drastic measures considered
- Positive inotropes (**DIGITALIS**, **MILRINONE**, $β_1$-agonists)
- Heart transplant
- Permanent mechanical support

NOTE: Additional terminology is also popular including:
- "Early Stage HF" (Stage C HF)
- "Progressive HF" (Stage C or Stage D HF where the patient needs positive inotropes including LOW dose cardiac glycosides)
- "End Stage HF" (Stage D where the patient needs HIGH doses of positive inotropes)

Take Home Point about Therapy

All stage B and some Stage C are treated with negative inotropes

Some stage C and all Stage D are treated with positive inotropes

Heart Failure: Negative Inotropes

> Negative inotropes are mainly used for Stage B and C heart failure

General Rules for Using β-blockers

1. Start and titrate slowly watching for side effects – rapid institution of β-blockers can precipitate decompensation
2. Add β-blockers at least two weeks after starting patient on ACE inhibitors (all Stage B and C patients must be on an ACE inhibitor)
3. Warn patient that symptoms of heart failure may get worse before they get better
4. β-adrenoceptors classified as β_1, β_2, and β_3 based on different drugs used to selectively stimulate or block each subtype
5. Some antagonists show greater selectivity for β_1-receptors in the heart: "cardioselective" (e.g. **METOPROLOL**, **ATENOLOL**)
   - Less likely to cause adverse effects of bronchospasm, intermittent claudication and cold extremities

Withdrawal of β-blockers

- Prolonged use of β-blockers leads to up-regulation of the receptor
- Abrupt cessation of therapy with β-blockers may cause exacerbation of angina or, in some cases, myocardial infarction
- Gradual withdrawal of β-blockers over 1-2 weeks is recommended

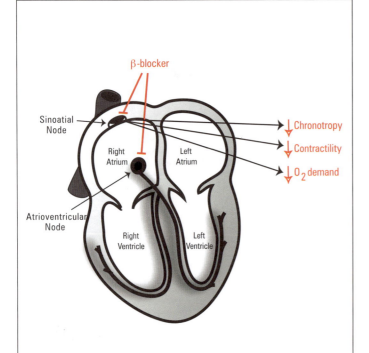

Figure 9. The Mechanism of Action of β-blockers in Heart Failure

METOPROLOL

MOA
- Decrease myocardial contractility and thereby decrease cardiac workload

USES
- Congestive heart failure (Stage B and Stage C)
- Angina

PK
- Short $t_{1/2}$ (3-4 hours)

ADRs

Side Effect	Caution for Patients with…
Bronchospasm	Asthma
Cardiodepression (bradycardia, heart block)	Stage D heart failure (specifically end stage heart failure), decreased contractility, bradycardia, 2nd/3rd degree heart block, untreated LV heart failure, heart failure patients with hypotension
Worsened PVD (uncompensated stimulation of α_1-mediated vasoconstriction by endogenous norepinephrine)	PVD
Hypoglycemia	Diabetics (particularly following insulin administration)
Fatigue, Depression	

DRUG INTERACTIONS

Agent	Effect
Antidiabetic agents	Hypoglycemia (β-antagonism in the liver and/or masking of hypoglycemic response)
Calcium channel blockers	Bradycardia, AV block, worsened heart failure
Cimetidine	Prolonging half-life of β-blocker
Clonidine	Hypertension during β-blocker withdraw (stop clonidine first)
Cyclosporine	Increased levels due to CYP inhibition
Digoxin	Potentiation of bradycardia
Rifampin	Lowered β-blocker levels due to CYP induction

Other β-blockers include:
BISOPROLOL (β_1) and **CARVEDILOL** (α_1, β_1, β_2)

CONTRAINDICATIONS
- Negative inotropes should not generally be used in the context of Stage D heart failure
- Caution in patients with new-onset acute decompensated heart failure; should not be treated with β-blockers until after they have stabilized for several days to weeks

NOTES
- β-blockers in general have both negative inotropic and negative chronotropic (decreased heart rate) effects
   - Used extensively in the treatment of hypertension, arrhythmia, and secondary prevention after myocardial infarction
   - Also used in thyrotoxicosis and glaucoma
- Ca^{2+}-channel blockers are negative inotropes, though less used in heart failure
   - Used to decrease blood pressure by decreasing cardiac contractility in conditions such hypertension
   - Decrease heart rate in the treatment of arrhythmia

Heart Failure: Positive Inotropes

Therapeutic Use of Inotropes

Positive Inotropes used only in Stage D heart failure or heart failure with chronic atrial fibrillation
- β-blockers are not used in the context of stage 4 CHF with volume overload

Positive Inotropes

Positive inotropes may worsen early stage congestive heart failure by increasing energy demands of the myocardium (excluding **DIGOXIN**).

PDE3 Inhibitors

MILRINONE

MOA
- Inhibits PDE3 → increased cAMP and PKA → amplification of β_1-agonist signal
- Ca^{2+} channel activation → improved contraction → increased cardiac output
- Phospholamban activation in sarcoplasmic reticulum → increased Ca^{2+} uptake → improved relaxation
- Vasodilation (via cGMP in blood vessels)

USES
- Short-term treatment of late stage CHF

PK
- Short $t_{1/2}$ (2 hours)
- Renal secretion

ADRs
- Arrhythmia, ventricular fibrillation
- Thrombocytopenia (bleeding)
- Headache
- Hypotension

NOTES
- Chronic therapy with **MILRINONE** has led to increased mortality

> **MILRINONE**
> Milro makes your platelets go
> Recall PDE5 and 6 are affected by **SILDENAFIL**

β₁-Agonist

DOBUTAMINE

MOA
- Synthetic derivative of dopamine
- Agonizes β_1 → increase cAMP and PKA
  - Ca^{2+} channel phosphorylated → increased Ca^{2+} influx → increased contraction (inotropy)
  - Phospholamban activation in sarcoplasmic reticulum → increased Ca^{2+} reuptake → improved relaxation (lusitropy)

USES
- Short-term/acute congestive heart failure (short-term because of β-receptor downregulation)

PK
- Very short $t_{1/2}$ (2 minutes)

ADRs
- Ventricular arrhythmia → sudden death (ventricular fibrillation) since β_1-receptors are expressed ubiquitously in the heart
- Excessive tachycardia
- Hypertension
- Dyspnea

DRUG INTERACTIONS
- **ISOCARBOXAZID**
- **LINEZOLID**

NOTES
- Tolerance may develop after prolonged use due to downregulation of β-receptors
  - Both β-agonists and nitrates have rapid development of resistance
- Patients on a β-blocker may have a decreased initial response to **DOBUTAMINE**

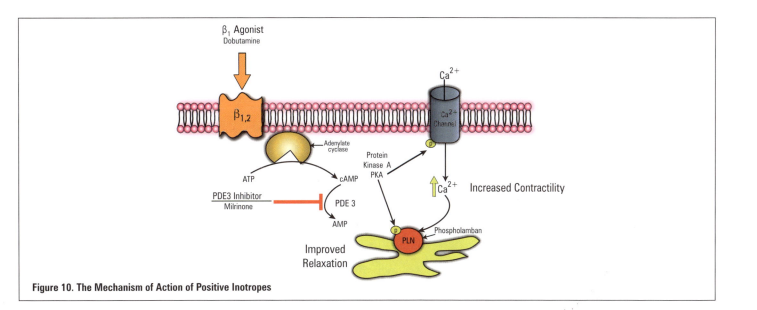

Figure 10. The Mechanism of Action of Positive Inotropes

Heart Failure: Cardiac Glycosides

Cardiac Glycosides (DIGOXIN and DIGITOXIN)
Mechanism of Action of Cardiac Glycosides

ENHANCED CARDIAC CONTRACTILITY
- By blocking Na+/K+ ATPase, the major path for shunting Na+ out of the myocyte is lost; increased intracellular Na+
- Na+/Ca2+ channel compensates for the high intracellular Na+ by reversing its normal direction of pumping: Na+ out of cell and Ca2+ into the cell
- Increased intracellular Ca2+ which enhances cardiac output and SV in 3 ways:
  - Increased myofilament contraction
  - Increased sarcoplasmic Ca2+ stores
  - Activated ryanodine receptor Ca2+ channel, increased Ca2+ release into cytosol

ENHANCED VAGAL "PARASYMPATHETIC" TONE
- Increase in intracellular Na+ in the presynaptic neuron results in the extracellular release of ACh which has 3 effects:
  - Increased ERP (refractoriness) in AV node
  - AV node increased ACh sensitivity → slower conduction to ventricle
  - Decreased catecholamine (NE, E, DA) sensitivity
- Increased baroreceptor sensitivity to vagal activity
- Increased muscarinic receptor sensitivity to acetylcholine (in atria)

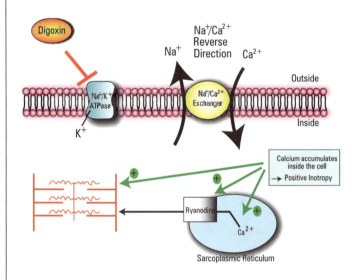

Figure 11. Enhancement of Contractility by Cardiac Glycosides

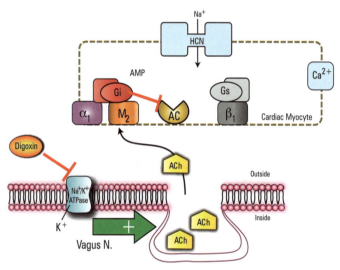

Figure 12. Enhancement of Vagal Tone by Cardiac Glycosides

DIGOXIN
USES
- Congestive heart failure
- Atrial fibrillation (slows ventricular response)
- Fetal supraventricular tachycardia (given to mother)

PK
- Very long $t_{1/2}$ (1-2 days)
- Renal elimination
- Bacteria (*Eubacterium*) in gut may inactivate DIGOXIN in 10% of population – antibiotics may be coadministered

CONTRAINDICATIONS
- Active myocardial ischemia
- Patients with pulmonary disease

ADRs
- Bradycardia
- Atrial tachycardia; AV block
- Hyperestrogenism – gynecomastia, galactorrhea, vaginal plaques
- Nausea, anorexia, vomiting
- Blurred vision, green/yellow halos around light
- Fatigue, muscle weakness, anxiety, nightmares, delirium

Cardiac Glycoside Toxicity

Digitalis intoxication is common (up to 25% of patients) because it has a low therapeutic index. Toxicity usually occurs in patients also taking diuretics (due to potassium loss). Toxicity can present with bradyarrhythmia (usually with acute toxicitiy and in younger persons) or tachycardia (usually in chronic toxicity and with existing heart disease).

Treatment of Digitalis Toxicity

KCl
- Restores serum K+ – both digitalis and K+ levels must be monitored carefully

DIGOXIN ANTIBODIES
- Fab fragments bind digitalis
- Used for life-threatening digitalis poisoning (especially if ventricular tachycardia and hyperkalemia are present)
- Can only use once per patient since can lead to serum sickness with second administration

Antihyperlipidemia Drugs

Introduction

Dietary and lifestyle modifications constitute the first-line treatment for hyperlipidemia. These measures, however, are often not enough to achieve ideal plasma lipid levels and so pharmacologic treatment is often necessary. Lipids are potentially atherogenic and a cholesterol level greater than 6.2 mmol/L (240 mg/dl) can double one's risk of coronary heart disease (CHD). The primary goals of the treatment of hyperlipidemia include reduction of cardiovascular disease risk, regression of atherosclerotic plaques, and elevation of HDL levels. HDLs retrieve cholesterol from blood vessel walls, preventing lipoprotein oxidation and thereby thwarting atherogenesis.

- Different antihyperlipidemic drugs have different efficacies for each of the various lipids:
  - Decreasing LDL levels:
    STATINS > RESINS = NIACIN > FIBRATES
  - Increasing HDL levels:
    NIACIN > STATINS = RESINS = FIBRATES
  - Decreasing TG levels:
    FIBRATES >> NIACIN = STATINS
    - NOTE that resins INCREASE TG levels!

- Risk factors (smoking, HTN, low HDL, familial CHD, men >45, women >55), for heart disease modify the goal blood levels of LDLs:
  - 1 risk factor → Goal LDL <160
  - 2+ risk factors → Goal LDL <130
  - CHD or CHD risk equivalents → Goal LDL <100

- Diabetes is a CHD risk equivalent, meaning that if you have diabetes, then your goal LDL is the same as if you have CHD (also abdominal aortic aneurysm and peripheral vascular disease)

- HDL >60 is protective against CHD, and is considered a negative risk factor

- Goal HDL is >40-60

Treatment of Dyslipidemia

Statins can reduce the risk of CHD events and nonhemorrhagic stroke in virtually every type of dyslipidemic patient. Statin therapy should be considered first-line for pharmacologic therapy. Target cholesterol levels should be determined and dose should be adjusted to obtain this target.

HMG-CoA Reductase Inhibitors

LOVASTATIN and **ATORVASTATIN**

MOA
- Competitively inhibits HMG-CoA reductase; reduced liver cholesterol concentration results and induces an upregulation of liver LDL receptors → resulting in decreased serum LDL
- Reduces inflammation, promoting regression of and reducing risk for rupture of atherosclerotic plaques
- Can reduce platelet aggregation

USES
- First-line drug for the treatment of hyperlipidemia
- Decreases LDL
- Reverses atherosclerosis
- Children heterozygous for familial hypercholesterolemia (must be able to express LDL receptors)

PK LOVASTATIN
- Significant first-pass metabolism by CYP in liver
- Hepatic metabolism to active metabolite
- Active metabolite has long $t_{1/2}$ (15 hours)

PK ATORVASTATIN
- Hepatic metabolism
- Long $t_{1/2}$ (14 hours)

ADRs
- Reversible elevation of liver enzymes
- Rhabdomyolysis or myositis (pain, elevated creatine kinase levels)
- Hepatotoxicity
- Abdominal pain, constipation, diarrhea, nausea
- Headache
- Myopathy

CONTRAINDICATIONS
- Liver disease
- Pregnancy and lactation

DRUG INTERACTIONS
- Heavy alcohol use may increase risk of liver disease
- Grapefruit juice
- Other drugs known to inhibit CYP

NOTES
- Peak response may require 4-6 weeks
- Statins act synergistically with bile acid binding resins
- **ATORVASTATIN** decreases both LDL and TGs
- Other examples include **ROSUVASTATIN**, **PRAVASTATIN**

Pancreatic Lipase Inhibitors

ORLISTAT

MOA
- Inhibition of pancreatic lipase; triglycerides are excreted from rather than metabolized in the gut

USES
- Only when patient is 30% or more overweight

PK
- Short $t_{1/2}$ (1-2 hours)

ADRs
- Steatorrhea (may cause deficiencies of vitamins A, D, E, K)
- Flatulence
- Frequent, uncontrollable bowel movements

CONTRAINDICATIONS
- Chronic malabsorptive disorders
- Gallbladder disease
- Pregnancy, breastfeeding

DRUG INTERACTIONS
- **CYCLOSPORINE**

Bile Acid Binding Resins

CHOLESTYRAMINE

MOA
- Binds to bile and prevents reabsorption in the ileum; reduced liver bile acid content drives bile acid synthesis from cholesterol, increasing liver LDL receptors
- Increases fecal excretion of bile acids

USES
- Treatment of elevated LDL
- NOT useful when LDL elevation is accompanied by hypertriglyceridemia (resin indirectly increases VLDL secretion)

PK
- Not absorbed; completely excreted in the feces

ADRs
- Steatorrhea (may cause deficiencies of vitamins A, D, E, K)
- Binding of other drugs in the GI tract (especially steroid-based drugs like **DIGITALIS**)

CONTRAINDICATIONS
- Biliary obstruction
- Type III, IV, or V hyperlipidemia

DRUG INTERACTIONS
- May inhibit absorption of other acidic drugs when taken concurrently
  - **WARFARIN**, barbiturates, **THYROXINE**, **DIGOXIN**

NOTES
- Compensatory VLDL secretion may result in increased TG levels
- Peak response may require 4 weeks
- Other bile acid binding resins include: **COLESTIPOL**

Antihyperlipidemia Drugs

NIACIN (Nicotinic acid; Vitamin B3)
MOA
- Exact mechanism unknown but thought to:
  - Inhibit VLDL secretion from the liver (to decrease VLDL)
  - Inhibit lipolysis in adipose tissue to decrease LDL
  - Reduce esterification of hepatic TGs
  - Increase HDL and reduce total cholesterol

USES
- Elevated VLDL and LDL
- Pellagra (niacin deficiency)

PK
- Extensive first pass metabolism
- Very short $t_{1/2}$ (20-45 minutes)

ADRs
- Pruritus (due to precipitation of cholesterol salts on skin)
- Cutaneous flush
  - Responsive to aspirin and ibuprofen (flushing is prostaglandin-mediated)
- Vasodilation, hypotension
- Dyspepsia
- Liver necrosis
- Hyperuricemia
- Myolysis

CONTRAINDICATIONS
- Liver disease
- Active peptic ulcer

DRUG INTERACTIONS
- Alcohol

NOTES
- Use with caution in diabetic patients since may result in insulin resistance

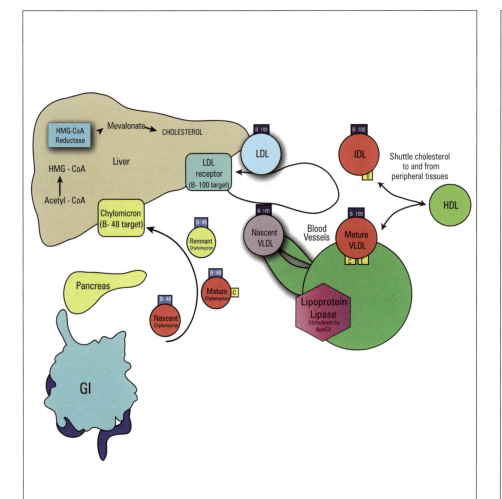

Figure 13. Antihyperlipidemia Drug Targets

Lipoprotein Lipase Stimulators (Fibrate Derivatives)

GEMFIBROZIL
MOA
- Decreases VLDL and increases HDL by unknown mechanism

USES
- Treatment of elevated VLDL (perturbation in dysbetalipoproteinemia)
- Familial type 5 hyperlipoproteinemia

PK
- Largely excreted unchanged by kidneys
- Short $t_{1/2}$ (1 hour)

ADRs
- Hypokalemia
- Gallbladder disease, gallstones
- Pruritus (due to precipitation of cholesterol salts on skin)
- Rhabdomyolysis (increased risk when statin is co-administered)
- Myoglobinuria (can lead to renal failure)

CONTRAINDICATIONS
- Biliary tract disease
- Hepatic dysfunction
- Severe renal impairment

DRUG INTERACTIONS
- Contraindicated with **REPAGLINIDE** – risk of hypoglycemia
- Statins
- **DIGOXIN** – exaggerates hypokalemia leading to fatal arrhythmia

NOTES
- Other fibrates include: **CLOFIBRATE**

Central Nervous System

Chapter Authors: Nicole C. Badie, Nicholas D. Boespflug, Amanda Carnevale, Robert B. Hufnagel, Monique Moller, Moumita Sarkar, Julianna L. Sienna, Margaret A. Stefater, Seth J. Stern and Inuk Zandvakili

Faculty Reviewers: Susan Belo, Yaron Finkelstein, Prateek Lala, Bernard Le Foll, Albert H.C. Wong and Cindy Woodland

IN THIS CHAPTER

Anti-Epileptic Drugs	75
Parkinson's Disease	76
Anesthetics	78
Local Anesthetics	
General Anesthetics – Inhaled	
General Anesthetics – Intravenous	
Analgesics	82
Non-Steroidal Anti-Inflammatory Drugs (NSAIDs)	
Aspirin	
Acetaminophen	
Opioids	
Benzodiazepines	86
Anti-Obesity Drugs	87
Antipsychotics	88
Mood Disorders	90
Antidepressants	
Mania	
Anxiolytics and Sedative-Hypnotics	93
Drugs of Abuse	95
Stimulants	
Opioids	
Nicotine	
Cannabinoids and Hallucinogens	
Dissociative Anesthetics	
Depressants and Volatile Inhalants	
Alcohol	
Alcohol Abuse and Dependence	

DRUGS IN THIS CHAPTER

Generic Name	US Trade Name	Canadian Trade Name
acamprosate	CAMPRAL	
acetaminophen	TYLENOL, GENAPAP, FEVERALL, ACTAMIN MAXIMUM STRENGTH, ALTENOL, AMINOFEN, ANACIN ASPIRIN FREE, APRA	ACET, ACETAZONE, ATASOL, TEMPRA, TYLENOL
alfentanil	ALFENTA	
alprazolam	XANAX, NIRAVAM, GABAZOLAMINE	ALPRAZ, XANAX
amantadine	SYMMETREL	AMANTADINE
amitriptyline	ELAVIL, VANATRIP	ELAVIL, TRIAVIL
aripiprazole	ABILIFY	
aspirin/ acetylsalicylic acid (ASA)	ECOTRIN, BAYER, ASCRIPTIN, ASPERGUM, ASPIRTAB, EASPRIN, ECPIRIN, ENTERCOTE	ASPIRIN
benztropine	COGENTIN	
bromocriptine	PARLODEL, CYCLOSET	PARLODEL
bupivacaine	MARCAINE, SENSORCAINE	
buprenorphine	BUTRANS, BUPRENEX, SUBUTEX	BUTRANS, SUBOXONE
bupropion	WELLBUTRIN, ZYBAN, BUDEPRION, BUPROBAN	WELLBUTRIN, ZYBAN
buspirone	BUSPAR, VANSPAR	BUSPAR, BUSTAB
carbamazepine	CARBATROL, EPITOL, TEGRETOL, EQUETRO	TEGRETOL
carbidopa	SINEMET, PARCOPA	LEVOCARB, PROLOPA, SINEMET, STALEVO
celecoxib	CELEBREX	
chloral hydrate	AQUACHLORAL SUPPRETTES, SOMNOTE	
chloroprocaine	NESACAINE	
chlorpromazine	THORAZINE	CHLORPROMANYL, LARGACTIL
citalopram	CELEXA	
clonazepam	KLONOPIN	RIVOTRIL
clozapine	CLOZARIL, FAZACLO	CLOZARIL
codeine		
dantrolene	DANTRIUM, REVONTO	DANTRIUM
desflurane	SUPRANE	
diazepam	DIASTAT, VALIUM	DIASTAT, DIAZAMULS, VALIUM

DRUGS IN THIS CHAPTER (continued)

Generic Name	US Trade Name	Canadian Trade Name
diphenhydramine	BENADRYL, DIPHENHIST, DIPHENYL, GENAHIST, GERIDRYL, NYTOL QUICKCAPS/QUICKGELS	ALLERDRYL, BALMINIL, BENADRYL, BENYLIN, BUCKLEY'S BEDTIME
diphenoxylate	LOMOCOT, LOMOTIL, LONOX, VI-ATRO	LOMOTIL
disulfiram	ANTABUSE	
doxylamine	UNISOM, ALDEX AN	DALMACOL, DICLECTIN, UNISOM
droperidol	INAPSINE	DROPERIDOL
entacapone	COMTAN	COMTAN, STALEVO
etomidate	AMIDATE	
fentanyl	DURAGESIC, ACTIQ, SUBLIMAZE, FENTORA, ONSOLIS, ABSTRAL	DURAGESIC
flumazenil	ROMAZICON	ANEXATE
fluoxetine	PROZAC, SARAFERN, RAPIFLUX, SELFERNRA	PROZAC
fluphenazine	PROLIXIN, PERMITIL, PROLIXIN DECANOATE	MODITEN, MODECATE
gabapentin	GABARONE, NEURONTIN, GRALISE	NEURONTIN
haloperidol	HALDOL	
halothane		
hydromorphone	DILAUDID, PALLADONE, EXALGO	DILAUDID, HYDROMORPH CONTIN, HYDROMORPH, JURNISTA
hydroxyzine pamoate	VISTARIL	ATARAX
ibuprofen	ADVIL, MOTRIN, A-G PROFEN, ADDAPRIN, BUFEN, GENPRIL, HALTRAN, I-PRIN	ADVIL, MOTRIN, PROFEN, PAMPRIN
imipramine	TOFRANIL	
indomethacin	INDOCIN	
isoflurane	FORANE, TERRELL	AERRANE, FORANE
ketamine	KETALAR	
ketorolac	ACULAR, TORADOL, ACUVAIL	ACULAR, TORADOL
lamotrigine	LARNICTAL	LAMICTAL
levodopa	SINEMET, PARCOPA	LEVOCARB, PROLOPA, SINEMET, STALEVO
loperamide	DIAMODE, IMODIUM, IMOGEN, IMOTIL, IMPERIM, KAO-PAVERIN CAPS, KAODENE A-D	IMODIUM, LOPERACAP
lorazepam	ATIVAN	
maprotiline	LUDIOMIL	
meperidine	DEMEROL, MEPERITAB	DEMEROL
methadone	DOLOPHINE, METHADOSE, DISKETS DISPERSIBLE	METADOL
methohexital	BREVITAL	BRIETAL
methoxyflurane	PENTHRANE	
midazolam	VERSED	
morphine	AVINZA, KADIAN, MS CONTIN, MS IR, ORAMORPH, ROXANOL, RMS	KADIAN, ESLON, MS CONTIN, MS IR, ORAMORPH, STATEX

Generic Name	US Trade Name	Canadian Trade Name
naloxone	NARCAN	NARCAN, TARGIN, SUBOXONE
naltrexone	VIVITROL, REVIA	REVIA
naproxen	NAPROSYN	
nitrous oxide		
normeperidine		
olanzapine	ZYPREXA	
oxycodone	DAZIDOX, ETH-OXYDOSE, OXYCONTIN, OXY IR, OXYDOSE, OXYFAST, ROXICODONE	ENDOCET, ENDODAN, OXYCONTIN, PERCOCET, SUPEUDOL, TARGIN (with naloxone)
paroxetine	PAXIL, PEXEVA	PAXIL
pentazocine	TALWIN	
pergolide	PERMAX	
phenelzine	NARDIL	
phenobarbital	LUMINAL	BELLERGAL SPACETABS, DONNATAL
phentermine	ADIPEX, ATTI-PLEX P, FASTIN, PHENTERCOT, PHENTRIDE, PRO-FAST, IONAMIN	IONAMIN
phenytoin	DILANTIN, PHENYTEK	DILANTIN
pramipexole	MIRAPEX	
prilocaine	CITANEST PLAIN DENTAL, EMLA, ORAQIX	EMLA CREAM/EMLA PATCH
procaine	CRYSTICILLIN, WYCILLIN	NOVOCAINE
propofol	DIPRIVAN, FRESENIOUS PROPOVEN	DIPRIVAN
quetiapine	SEROQUEL	
risperidone	RISPERDAL	
rofecoxib	VIOXX	
ropinirole	REQUIP	
ropivacaine	NAROPIN	
selegiline	EMSAM, ELDEPRYL, ZELAPAR	ELDEPRYL
sertraline	ZOLOFT	
sevoflurane	ULTANE, SOJOURN	SEVORANE
thiopental	PENTOTHAL	
tolcapone	TASMAR	
topiramate	TOPAMAX, TOPIRAGEN	TOPAMAX
tramadol	ULTRAM, RYZOLT, RYBIX ODT	RALIVIA, TRAMACET, TRIDURAL, ULTRAM, ZYTRAM
tranylcypromine	PARNATE	
trazodone	DESYREL, OLEPTRO	DESYREL, TRAZOREL
tubocurarine		
valproate	DEPAKENE, STAVZOR	DEPAKENE, DEPROIC
varenicline	CHANTIX	CHAMPIX
venlafaxine	EFFEXOR	
zaleplon	SONATA	STARNOC
zolpidem	AMBIEN, EDLUAR, ZOLPIMIST	

Anti-Epileptic Drugs

Seizure – abnormal, hypersynchronous discharge of cortical neurons

Clinical Seizure – produce subjective symptoms and apparent signs

Electrographic Seizure – only visible on EEG

Epilepsy is the disorder of recurring seizures (not just one seizure)

SEIZURE TYPES
- **Partial/Focal:** arises from one part of the brain
  - **Simple:** no loss of consciousness
  - **Complex:** loss of consciousness
- Treatment:
  - CARBAMAZAPINE, PHENYTOIN, GABAPENTIN, LAMOTRIGINE, TOPIRAMATE, VALPROATE

- **Generalized:** abnormal activity in entire brain
  - **Primary:** Seizure activity begins as generalized
  - **Secondary:** Seizure progresses from partial to generalized
- Treatment:
  - VALPROATE, PHENYTOIN, CARBAMAZAPINE, LAMOTRIGINE, TOPIRAMATE, GABAPENTIN, PHENOBARBITAL

- **Status Epilepticus:** unrelenting seizure state
- Treatment:
  - PHENYTOIN, BENZODIAZEPINES

- Mono-AED therapy is preferred
- AEDs in combination rarely benefit patients

Antiepileptic Drugs (AED)
- All antiepileptic drugs have similar efficacy
- NOTE: Children metabolize the drugs more rapidly

Pregnancy and AED & Epilepsy Guidelines
- 2-3 fold increase in birth defects
- Maternal seizures may be deleterious to the fetus
- All pregnant women using AEDs should supplement with folic acid
- Counselling with a teratogen information service is recommended

Na+ Channel Inactivators

PHENYTOIN
ADRs
- Gingival hypertrophy
- Ataxia
- Diplopia
- Nystagmus
- Hirsuitism
- Megaloblastic anemia
- Lupus

LAMOTRIGINE
ADRs
- Stevens-Johnson Syndrome

CARBAMAZAPINE
ADRs
- Ataxia
- Diplopia
- Aplastic anemia
- Hepatotoxicity

Ca²⁺ Channel Inhibitor

ETHOSUXIMIDE
ADRs
- Stevens-Johnson Syndrome
- GI distress
- Urticaria
- Headache

GABA Augmenters

BENZODIAZEPINES

VALPROATE
(also increases Na+ channel inactivation)

ADRs
- Weight gain
- Tremor
- Alopecia
- GI distress
- Hepatotoxicity

TOPIRAMATE
(also blocks Na+ channels)

ADRs
- Mental dullness
- Weight loss
- Kidney stones

GABAPENTIN
ADRs
- Ataxia

PHENOBARBITAL
ADRs
- Dependence
- Respiratory and cardiovascular depresion

NOTES
- Not teratogenic

Parkinson's Disease

While the etiology for Parkinson's Disease (PD) is unknown, it is established that PD arises as a result of the degeneration of dopaminergic neurons in the substantia nigra pars compacta, which form the nigrostriatal dopamine pathway. This leads to imbalanced dopaminergic and cholinergic transmission; accordingly, pharmacologic therapy for Parkinson's patients is targeted toward these two neurotransmitter systems. Enhancing dopaminergic function is the main approach, while inhibition of cholinergic function is an alternative but less effective approach to PD treatment. Current pharmacological treatment of PD is palliative only, and targets the major and often debilitating symptoms: bradykinesia, muscle tremor and rigidity ("cogwheel rigidity"), and postural impairment. Non-pharmacologic therapies in use and in development include pallidotomy, deep brain stimulation, and neuronal grafts.

The current therapy of choice for PD is a combination of **L-DOPA** and **CARBIDOPA**. **L-DOPA** is a synthetic dopamine (DA) derivative, which is unique in its ability to cross the blood-brain barrier. In the CNS, **L-DOPA** is converted to DA, thereby replenishing nigrostriatal DA availability. However, **L-DOPA** administration alone results in minimal penetration of active concentrations into the CNS, as much of the drug is rapidly metabolized before reaching systemic circulation. Additionally, significant peripheral **L-DOPA** concentrations often lead to undesired adverse effects. **CARBIDOPA** inhibits peripheral metabolism of **L-DOPA**, thereby boosting the CNS effects of **L-DOPA** without exacerbating the peripherally-mediated side effects of the drug.

Other drugs are generally used as adjuncts to this first-line combination therapy and generally do not replace an **L-DOPA** plus carbidopa regimen. These drugs may be used to try to increase the usefulness of **L-DOPA/CARBIDOPA** by minimizing **L-DOPA/CARBIDOPA** sensitivity that arises from prolonged administration.

It is important to remember not to treat a Parkinson's patient with any antidopaminergic drug. Although drugs for other diseases may target extrastriatal dopaminergic neurotransmission, all antidopaminergic drugs are fairly nonspecific and therefore may exacerbate the motor problems caused by PD. Drugs to be avoided include tricyclic antidepressants, certain anti-emetics (**METOCLOPRAMIDE**, **DOMPERIDONE**) and atypical antipsychotics.

L-DOPA (Levodopa)

MOA
- Converted via decarboxylation to DA in CNS
- Largely ineffective if administered without inhibitor of peripheral metabolism, e.g. **CARBIDOPA**

USES
- First line treatment of PD

PK
- **L-DOPA**: Short $t_{1/2}$ (0.75-1.5 hours)
- Increases after co-administration with **CARBIDOPA** (1.5-2 hours)

ADRs
- Dyskinesia (dose-dependent and reversible)
- Hypotension
- Nausea
- GI distress

CONTRAINDICATIONS
- MAO inhibitors

NOTES
- "Wearing off" phenomenon: degree of improvement after given dose decreases over time
- Increased dosing frequency may elevate risk for ADRs
- "On/off" phenomenon: after chronic administration, patients may fluctuate between experiencing therapeutic effects and phases of immobility

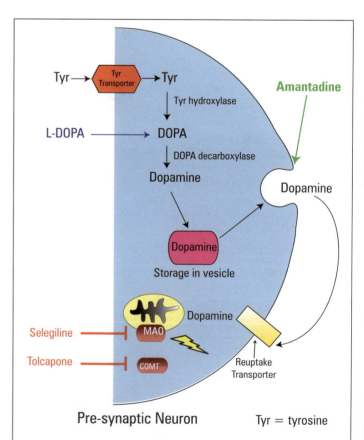

Figure 1A. Mechanism of Action of Therapeutics to Treat Parkinson's Disease

Parkinson's Disease

PERGOLIDE, PRAMIPEXOLE, ROPINIROLE, BROMOCRIPTINE

MOA
- Direct agonists of post-synaptic DA receptors
  - All active at D_2, only **PERGOLIDE** and **BROMOCRIPTINE** (partial agonist) active at D_1

USES
- Preferred as initial treatment in younger PD cases

PK
- **PERGOLIDE**
  - Long $t_{1/2}$ (~27 hours)
- **PRAMIPEXOLE**
  - Long $t_{1/2}$ (8-12 hours)
- **ROPINIROLE**
  - Moderate $t_{1/2}$ (~6 hours)
- **BROMOCRIPTINE**
  - Long $t_{1/2}$ (12-14 hours)

ADRs
- Hypotension
- Hallucinosis or confusion

NOTES
- Newer agents (**PRAMIPEXOLE, ROPINIROLE**) are preferred due to higher selectivity for D_2 receptors

AMANTADINE

MOA
- Activates presynaptic DA release

USES
- Modest effects in early PD
- Reduces dyskinesia

PK
- Long $t_{1/2}$ (~17 hours)

ADRs
- Anticholinergic effects
- Nervousness and anxiety
- Insomnia

SELEGILINE

MOA
- Selective and irreversible inhibition of MAO-B (only found in CNS)
  - Decreases metabolism of DA

USES
- Modest effects in early PD
- May provide neuroprotective effect

PK
- Oral: Short $t_{1/2}$ (~1 hour)
- Transdermal: Long $t_{1/2}$ (18-25 hours)

ADRs
- May enhance adverse effects of **L-DOPA**
- Sympathomimetic stimulatory effects (metabolites include amphetamine)

DRUG INTERACTIONS
- MAO inhibitors
- SSRIs
- Tyramine-rich foods

TOLCAPONE, ENTACAPONE

MOA
- Inhibits COMT, enzyme responsible for metabolism of **L-DOPA** and DA

USES
- Used in adjunct with **L-DOPA** therapy

PK
- **TOLCAPONE** – Short $t_{1/2}$ (1.5-3 hours)
- **ENTACAPONE** – Short $t_{1/2}$ (1-2 hours)

ADRs
- Dyskinesia (dose-dependent and reversible)
- Hypotension
- Nausea
- Hepatotoxicity (**TOLCAPONE** only)

BENZTROPINE

MOA
- Muscarinic receptor antagonist

USES
- Improvement of tremor
- Less effective for rigidity and bradykinesia
- Useful in treatment of early PD

PK
- Short $t_{1/2}$ (2-3 hours)

ADRs
- Anticholinergic effects
- Psychosis (dose-dependent)

CONTRAINDICATIONS
- Narrow-angle glaucoma

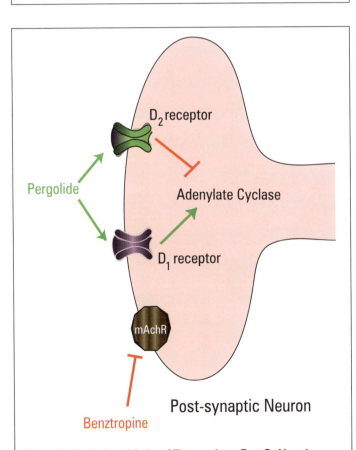

Figure 1B. Mechanism of Action of Therapeutics to Treat Parkinson's Disease

Anesthetics

Anesthetics may be used for either local sensory nerve block or to induce loss of consciousness in the patient. Anesthesia refers to the loss of all sensory input and is distinct from analgesia (pain relief). For each of the following drug classes, drug lipophilicity and solubility are important because these properties determine the compartmentalization of the drug. Another key concept to note is drug potency and, in particular, the concept of minimum alveolar content (MAC) for inhaled general anesthetics.

Anesthetics are divided into two classes:
- **Local anesthetics (LA)** are usually applied topically or injected locally. The pH of a local anesthetic affects its ability to enter a neuron and alter sodium channel excitability
- **General anesthetics (GA)** may be injected directly into systemic circulation or inhaled. The solubility of a general anesthetic drug in the blood affects both the speed of induction and recovery in response to the drug

Local Anesthetics

MOA (For all LAs)
- Block voltage-gated sodium channels that typically respond to depolarization of membrane
  - Inhibit propagation of action potential and, consequently, nerve conduction
- LAs bind only to channels in open or inactive state, holding channel in the inactive state and preventing flow of ions through the channel
- Block channels/neurons with high-firing frequency, and long action potential duration
- Thin axons are blocked more rapidly than thick axons
- LAs block pain and autonomic nerve fibers first:
  - Narrow diameter
  - Slow conduction velocity

All LAs are weak bases
- Uncharged drug molecules can cross cell membranes
- Once inside cell, acidic pH ionizes and traps drug (ion trapping)
- Avoids diffusion into neighbouring regions

Increased LA lipid solubility means:
- Increased potency
- Faster action
- Increased duration of action

Rate of systemic absorption depends on:
- Tissue vasculature
- Rate of metabolism
  - Ester-type LAs are metabolized in the blood
  - Amide-type LAs are metabolized in the liver
- Tissue pH

ORDER OF BLOCK BY SYSTEM (occurs when LA enters systemic circulation)
1. CNS (tingling, vision, hearing)
2. PNS (shivering, twitching, tonic clonic seizure)
3. Cardiovascular (bradycardia, hypotension)

ORDER OF NERVE BLOCK
1. Pain
2. Autonomic
3. Temperature
4. Touch
5. Deep Pressure
6. Motor

RANK OF TOXICITY
1. Chloroprocaine (least)
2. Prilocaine
3. Procaine
4. Lidocaine
5. Ropivacaine
6. Bupivacaine (most)

Central Administration of Local Anesthetics

EPIDURAL ANESTHESIA
- Inject around dura and arachnoid matres

Advantages
- Multiple repeat dosing is possible via continuous epidural catheter
- Better control over spread of anesthesia
- Lower risk of hypotension

Disadvantages
- More technically challenging placement than spinal anesthesia
- Possible local anesthetic toxicity especially in repeated dosing schemes

SPINAL (AKA SUBARACHNOID OR INTRATHECAL) ANESTHESIA
- Anesthetic injected into CSF
- Technically easier procedure than epidural analgesia

Disadvantages
- Hypotension
- Inability to control the spread of anesthesia
- Possibility of post-dural puncture headache (PDPH)

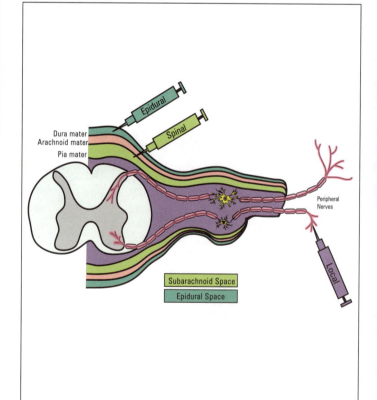

Figure 2. Administration Sites for Local Anesthetics

Local Anesthetics

Ester Type

- Rapidly metabolized in plasma by pseudocholinesterase
  - Shorter half-life/duration
- **Contraindicated in patients with sulfa drug allergies**
  - All ester types are metabolized to a PABA metabolite
- Cocaine, Tetracaine, Benzocaine are also ester type

CHLOROPROCAINE
USES
- Minor surgery
- Obstetric delivery (rapid metabolism prevents toxic levels from accumulating in the fetus)
- Infiltration
- Peripheral nerve block

PK
- Very short $t_{1/2}$ (~25 seconds)

ADRs
- **Neurotoxicity** (with older preparations)
- Muscular back pain (following epidural)

NOTES
- Fast onset
- Short (15-30 minutes) duration
- Most quickly metabolized local anesthetic

PROCAINE
USES
- Infiltration (main use)
- Spinal anesthesia

NOTES
- Slow onset
- Short duration

Amide Type

- Slowly metabolized in the liver
  - Longer half-life/duration

LIDOCAINE
USES
- Infiltration
- IV local anesthetic
- Peripheral nerve block
- Obstetric epidural
- Spinal anesthesia
- Topical anesthesia

NOTES
- Fast onset
- Medium (1-2 hours) duration
- Most commonly used medium-duration local anesthetic

PRILOCAINE
USES
- Infiltration
- IV local anesthesia
- Peripheral nerve block
- Epidural (NOT obstetric)

NOTES
- Little vasodilation, thus can use without epinephrine
- Most quickly metabolized amide

ROPIVACAINE
USES
- Infiltration
- Peripheral nerve block
- Obstetric epidural
- Spinal anesthesia

NOTES
- Medium onset
- Long (4-6 hours) duration

BUPIVACAINE
USES
- Infiltration
- Peripheral nerve block
- Obstetric epidural
- Spinal anesthesia

ADRs
- Highly cardiotoxic

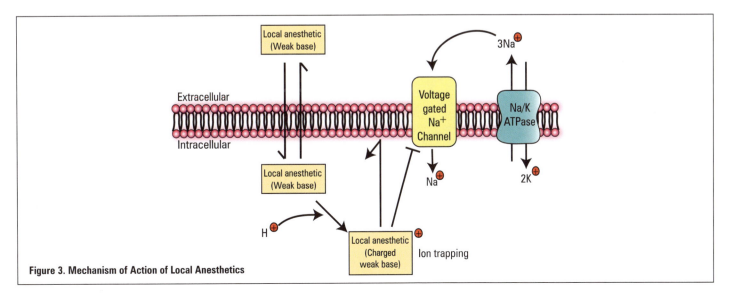

Figure 3. Mechanism of Action of Local Anesthetics

General Anesthetics – Inhaled

Notes

MAC= **M**inimum **A**lveolar **C**oncentration
- Concentration of anesthetic which produces unresponsiveness in 50% of patients exposed to a surgical procedure or painful stimuli while under anesthesia
- Potency is inversely related to MAC
  - High MAC = low potency (least toxic)
  - Low MAC = high potency (most toxic)
- MACs for coadministered drugs are additive
  e.g. 0.5 N_2O + 0.5 halothane = 1.0 total

	MACs (%)	Blood:Gas Partition Coefficient at 37°C
Methoxyflurane	0.2	10-14
Halothane	0.75	2.3
Isoflurane	1.2	1.4
Enflurane	1.6	1.8
Sevoflurane	2.0	0.65
Desflurane	6.0	0.45
Nitrous Oxide (N_2O)	105.0	0.47

Potency does NOT necessarily determine induction
- Induction is determined by the blood:gas partition coefficient
  - Low blood:gas = faster induction
  - High blood:gas = slower induction
- Children – ventilation is more significant than cardiac output → faster induction
- Rapid minute ventilation increases dose delivery of drug → faster induction
- Higher cardiac output → slower rise in alveolar partial pressure → slower induction

- Physiology affects MAC value for a given drug:

Decreased MAC	Increased MAC
Old age	Children
Hypothermia	Hyperthermia
Anemia	Tolerance
Hypotension	
Narcotics/premedicate	

Drugs with lower blood solubility cause quicker induction and quicker recovery
- A drug that is relatively insoluble in blood tends to move quickly from the blood into tissue

MOA
- Target is unknown
- Likely involves interactions with multiple receptor sites to interfere with synaptic transmissions
- All increase respiration rate and decrease total ventilation

USES
- Anesthetic – Induction and maintenance (**HALOTHANE** = gold standard)
- **N_2O** – Analgesic
- **SEVOFLURANE** – Mask induction, ambulatory surgery (quick recovery)

ADRs
- Myocardial depression
- Respiratory depression
- Hypotension – except **N_2O**
- Nausea/vomiting
- Increased cerebral blood flow
- Malignant hyperthermia
  - Most commonly observed with the combination of **HALOTHANE** and **SUCCINYLCHOLINE**
  - Use **DANTROLENE** to treat

DRUGS WITH A FLUORIDE ION METABOLITE ARE THE MOST TOXIC
- If highly metabolized then it is likely to be toxic because of fluoride metabolite; all are fluranes except **N_2O** and **HALOTHANE**

PK
- Steep dose response curves (high sensitivity)
- Tissue perfusion determines saturation and effect
  - Highly perfused organs: brain, heart, liver, kidney
  - Intermediate perfusion: skin and muscle
  - Low perfusion: fat, bone, tendon, connective tissue

ISOFLURANE, DESFLURANE

ADRs
- Increase HR
- Irritated airways
- Laryngospasm
- Breath holding
- Uterine relaxation
- Neurodegeneration in young children

CONTRAINDICATIONS
- Not suitable for pediatric induction (use IV induction instead)

NOTES (ISOFLURANE)
- Potentiates non depolarizing neuromuscular blockade
- Faster induction/recovery than halothane

ENFLURANE

ADRs
- Seizures (especially in children)

CONTRAINDICATIONS
- Contraindicated in patients with an abnormal EEG or a seizure disorder (**ENFLURANE** causes abnormal EEGs)
- **ENFLURANE** is not commonly used in pediatric anesthesia, because of seizure risk

NOTES
- Greater muscle relaxation than halothane

SEVOFLURANE

NOTES
- Excellent depth control
- Rapid recovery

HALOTHANE

ADRs
- Decrease heart rate
- Arrhythmia (due to sensitization to catecholamines)
- Increased intracranial pressure
- Decreased renal perfusion
- Halothane hepatitis
- Malignant hyperthermia

INTERACTIONS
- Concomitant use of other depressants, e.g. barbiturates, narcotics, may lead to additive effects
- **HALOTHANE** – do not use with drugs that increase catecholamines in the synapse (e.g. TCAs)

NITROUS OXIDE (N_2O)

ADRs
- Expands pockets of gas in body (abdomen, chest, skull)
- Decreased leukocyte/RBC production
- Megaloblastic bone marrow changes
- Irreversibly oxidizes vitamin B_{12} which may lead to vitamin B_{12} deficiency

NOTES
- Least toxic general inhalational anesthetic
- No scent

METHOXYFLURANE

ADRs
- Nephrotoxicity from fluoride ions produced by renal metabolism

NOTES
- Not widely used (slow acting, long lasting)
- Long recovery

General Anesthetics – Intravenous

GABA Receptor Agonists

Ultrashort Acting Barbiturates

MOA
- $GABA_A$ receptor agonists, increased duration of channel opening
- GABA independent

USES
- Anesthesia only
  (no analgesia or skeletal muscle relaxation)
- Unconsciousness
- Amnesia
- May be supplemented with N_2O or an opioid analgesic

ADRs
- Transient drop in blood pressure
  (due to vasodilation)
- Cardiovascular depression
  (decreased contractility)
- Respiratory depression
- Hypersensitivity reaction
- Sedation

THIOPENTAL
- Short duration surgical procedure

METHOHEXITAL
- 2X shorter duration and faster recovery than thiopental
- 3X more potent than thiopental

Short Acting Benzodiazepines

MIDAZOLAM

MOA
- $GABA_A$ receptor agonists, increased frequency of channel opening
- GABA dependent – GABA must also be present to activate $GABA_A$

USES
- Used in high doses for anesthesia
- Endoscopy
- Unconsciousness without analgesia

ADRs
- Anterograde amnesia
- Severe post-operative respiratory depression and amnesia
- Less cardiovascular and respiratory depression than barbiturates
- Benzodiazepine overdose may be reversed with **FLUMAZENIL** (GABA receptor antagonist)

PK
- Rapid induction
- Very lipid soluble → crosses membranes easily → enters CNS
- Drug distribution over time is dependent upon tissue vascularization
- Highly vascularized tissues receive more drug initially
- Short-acting drugs are short-acting due to redistribution, not metabolism
- If cardiac output is reduced, drug will be more slowly redistributed and reduced clearance from the site of action (CNS)

Notes
- No GAs offer analgesia except **KETAMINE, ALFENTANIL**

PROPOFOL

MOA
- Increased inhibition via $GABA_A$ receptors

USES
- Rapid induction
- Short procedures (rapid recovery)

ADRs
- Transient LARGE reduction in blood pressure due to peripheral vasodilation
- Transient apnea
- Pain on injection

CONTRAINDICATIONS
- Pre-medicated with opioids
- Patients with heart disease because of blood pressure effects

ETOMIDATE

MOA
- Ultra short acting non-barbiturate hypnotic agent acting at reticular-activating system
- Binds $GABA_A$ receptor, increases duration of chloride channel opening → increased post-synaptic effect of GABA → inhibition

USES
- Anesthesia without analgesia
- When it is necessary to:
  - Preserve cardiac output
  - Preserve respiratory stability

ADRs
- Hypotension, nausea, vomiting in recovery

KETAMINE

MOA
- NMDA receptor antagonist

USES
- Dissociative anesthesia
- Sedation, immobility, amnesia
- Delirient
- Analgesia

ADRs
- Disorientation, hallucination, nightmares
- Cardiovascular stimulation

NOTES
- Does NOT cause:
  - Generalized relaxation
  - Respiratory depression
  - Loss of airway reflexes

ALFENTANIL

MOA
- Opioid analgesic
- Decreases intracellular cAMP by inhibiting adenylate cyclase → inhibit neurotransmitter release
- Analgesic activity due to its conversion to morphine
- Hyperpolarization → reduced neuronal excitability

USES
- Anesthesia at high dose
- Cardiovascular surgery because minimal cardiovascular depression
- Only IV GA used for major invasive procedures
- Analgesia

ADRs
- Severe respiratory depression
- Pinpoint pupils
- Increased intracranial pressure
- Severe sedation
- Reversal with **NALOXONE**

DROPERIDOL

MOA
- Neuroleptic – mechanism unknown

USES
- Neuroleptanesthesia (patient is conscious and communicative but completely disinterested and detached)
- Antiemetic
- Antifibrillatory
- Anticonvulsant

ADRs
- Malignant neuroleptic syndrome

Analgesics

Non-Steroidal Anti-Inflammatory Drugs (NSAIDs)

NSAIDs are a class of drugs that are not chemically related but inhibit cyclooxygenase (COX) enzyme activity. Drugs that inhibit COX activity are collectively referred to as non-steroidal anti-inflammatory drugs (NSAIDs) and have beneficial effects that warrant their use in a variety of clinical scenarios. COX isoforms are expressed in all tissues, as such, there are a variety of negative outcomes to NSAID use (adverse drug reactions).

Unlike other NSAIDs, aspirin irreversibly inhibits COX. Therefore, when aspirin interacts with COX, new COX protein needs to be synthesized to restore activity.

Leukotriene and prostaglandin (PG) mediated signaling are regulated by lipoxygenase and COX enzymes, respectively. This balance is particularly important to aspirin induced asthma. Furthermore, different isoforms of COX (COX-1 and COX-2) are expressed in different cell types, yielding different outcomes to their inhibition.

- **Irreversible** COX inhibitors: Aspirin
- **Reversible** COX inhibitors: Ibuprofen
- Slower, **time-dependent** COX inhibitors: Indomethacin, Flurbiprofen
- **COX-2 selective** inhibitors: Celecoxib

NOTES
- Pharmacokinetics of NSAIDs
  - Rapid extensive oral absorption
  - Mostly liver metabolism
  - Highly protein bound, so poorly removed by dialysis

IBUPROFEN, NAPROXEN, INDOMETHACIN, KETOROLAC
MOA
- REVERSIBLE inhibition of COX-1 and COX-2

USES
- **Antipyretic**
  - Decreases medullary set point centrally and helps vascular dilation peripherally
- **Anti-inflammatory**
  - Via PGE2 inhibition
- **Analgesic**
  - Blocking PGs, blocks up-regulation of bradykinin receptors
- **DOC**
  - **KETOROLAC** for urgent pain due to its IV and IM formulations
  - **INDOMETHACIN** for acute gouty pain and for closure of patent ductus arteriosus
  - **NAPROXEN** when infrequent dosing desired ($t_{1/2}$ ~8-12 hours)

ADRs (primarily mediated via PG inhibition)
- **Renal injury, acute interstitial nephritis**
  - Decreased renal blood flow; increased concentrations of renally excreted drugs
- Gastric upset and ulceration (specifically antral ulcers)
  - Via PGI_2 inhibition which decreases acid regulation and mucous production
- Platelet dysfunction, rare aplastic anemia
  - Decreased aggregation secondary to platelet inability to form Thromboxane 2
- Slows labor and parturition
  - By decreasing PGs that help with cervical contractions
- Uricosuric
  - At low doses: blocks uric acid secretion
  - At high doses >5 g: blocks uric acid reabsorption
- Nausea and emesis
  - Chemoreceptor zone stimulation

CONTRAINDICATIONS
- **VERY IMPORTANT**
  - RENAL FAILURE, LIVER IMPAIRMENT, RENAL INSUFFICIENCY, drug allergy
- **Relative contraindications**
  - Peptic ulcer disease, GERD, bleeding disorders
- Pregnancy (3rd trimester, may close ductus arteriosus)

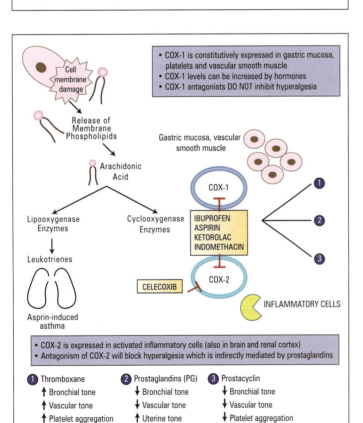

Figure 4. Mechanism of Action of Cyclooxygenase Inhibitors

COX-2 Inhibitors

CELECOXIB
MOA
- Reversible inhibition of COX-2 (found in inflammatory cells)

USES
- Anti-inflammatory

ADRs
- Cerebral ischemia
- Increased risk of thrombosis

CONTRAINDICATIONS
- Sulfa allergy

Analgesics

Aspirin (Acetylsalicylic Acid or ASA)

Differs from other NSAIDs because of its irreversible effects on thromboxane, which is a protein that cannot be replaced in platelets.

MOA
- **IRREVERSIBLE** cyclooxygenase inhibition (COX-1 and -2)
- Decreases formation of precursors of thromboxane and prostaglandins (PGs) from arachidonic acid
- Inhibits prostaglandin cyclooxygenase in platelets → prevents formation of thromboxane A2

USES
- **Anticoagulant** – secondary prevention of
  - Stroke
  - Myocardial infarction
  - Management of intermittent claudication
- Antipyretic and analgesic
- Anti-inflammatory

PK
- Hydrolyzed in liver to salicylic acid, conjugated and excreted in urine
- Half-life increases with greater dosage; first order elimination at therapeutic doses, zero order elimination at higher doses
  - Aspirin
    - Very short $t_{1/2}$ (15 minutes)
  - Salicylate (aspirin metabolite)
    - Short $t_{1/2}$ (2-3 hours)

ADRs
- Common
  - GI: nausea, vomiting, cramps, heartburn
  - Increased prothrombin time
  - Hypersensitivity – ↑ leukotriene synthesis → bronchoconstriction
  - **ASPIRIN**-induced asthma
    - Caused by the increase in leukotriene synthesis secondary to COX-inhibition
- Rare
  - GI ulceration
    - Pyloric, duodenal and particularly antral
  - Reye's syndrome
    - May occur when given to children during acute viral infection, such as chicken pox or influenza
  - Ototoxicity (tinnitus, vertigo)

DRUG INTERACTIONS
- Anticoagulants
  - Increased bleeding tendency

CONTRAINDICATIONS
- Not to be used in children with febrile disease due to the risk of developing Reye's syndrome: encephalopathy and fatty hepatic degradation
- Alcohol

NOTES
- **ASPIRIN** overdose or toxicity can be classified by severity:
  - **Mild** (non-systemic effects)
    - Emesis, erythema, gastritis
  - **Moderate** (systemic non-life threatening)
    - CNS stimulation, hyperpnea, mild combined anion-gap acidosis, tinnitus, hyperthermia-due to uncoupling of oxidative phosphorylation, coagulopathy
  - **Severe** (life-threatening); dosage varies by age and other factors
    - Ketolactic metabolic acidosis with respiratory alkalosis, seizure, hemorrhagic gastritis, CNS depression: lethargy, coma, death

Treatment of ASPIRIN toxicity
- GI decontamination – activated charcoal recommended if 2 hours within ingestion
- Once absorbed completely – dialysis
- Alkalinizing urine – promotes excretion of salicylic acids

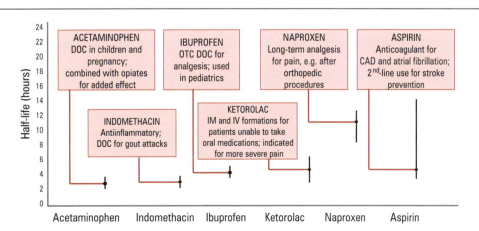

Figure 5. The Half-lives of Several Common Non-narcotic Analgesics

Analgesics

Acetaminophen

ACETAMINOPHEN (APAP), or **PARACETAMOL**, falls under the class of aniline analgesics. It is an over-the-counter medication used in the relief of headaches, fever, and mild-to-moderate pain. It is used in a variety of medications to treat cold- and flu-related symptoms, and is often combined with opioids for the treatment of more significant pain. The anti-inflammatory activity of APAP is insignificant, and thus, it is relatively ineffective in the treatment of inflammatory conditions. APAP is commonly used since it is well-tolerated and lacks notable adverse reactions at therapeutic doses. Unfortunately, its prevalence has lead to frequent incidences of hepatic injury as a result of both accidental and intentional overdoses.

ACETAMINOPHEN
MOA
- Central inhibition of prostaglandin synthetase → selectively inhibits COX-2

USES
- Anti-pyretic
- Analgesic (combined with opiates for added effect)
- **DOC in infants and during pregnancy**

PK
- Short $t_{1/2}$ (2-4 hours)

ADRs
- **LIVER: Hepatotoxicity** (dose-dependent)
- Occurs more often in alcoholics and when patients take more than recommended dose
  - Max dose of 4 g/day
  - 3.2 g/day chronic use
  - 2.4 g/day in elderly
  - 90 mg/kg/day in children
- Renal toxicity

CONTRAINDICATIONS
- Liver pathology: hepatitis, elevated liver enzymes
- Chronic alcohol consumption

NOTES
- **ACETAMINOPHEN** is not technically an NSAID and has negligible anti-inflammatory effects, and negligible antiplatelet activity

Acetaminophen Toxicity

- When the liver is unburdened, it can safely excrete acetaminophen (APAP) by conjugating approximately half the drug into glucuronate, another third into sulfonates and a small amount into cysteine and mercaptopurines by utilizing glutathione
- When APAP toxicity occurs, glutathione depletion results in ↑'d toxic metabolite
- Briefly, hepatic necrosis in toxicity occurs via glutathione depletion when toxic metabolite covalently binds to liver cells

TREATMENT OF TOXICITY
- Rumack-Matthew nomogram: used to estimate likelihood/extent of hepatic damage and helps guide the caregiver in treatment measures
- Oral or IV N-acetylcysteine given within the first 15 hours stabilizes APAP intermediate metabolite and prevents glutathione depletion
- Activated charcoal can be given in early or massive ingestions to prevent further absorption of the drug from the gut

Four Phases of Acetaminophen Toxicity

1. **First phase (0-24 hours)**
   - Often asymptomatic
   - May involve nausea, vomiting, sweating
2. **Second phase (24-72 hours)**
   - Elevation in hepatic enzymes, increased INR
   - Abdominal tenderness around liver
3. **Third phase (72-96 hours)**
   - Hepatic necrosis, encephalopathy, coma, renal failure, death
4. **Fourth phase (92+ hours)**
   - Surviving patients will have complete resolution of symptoms with no permanent liver injury

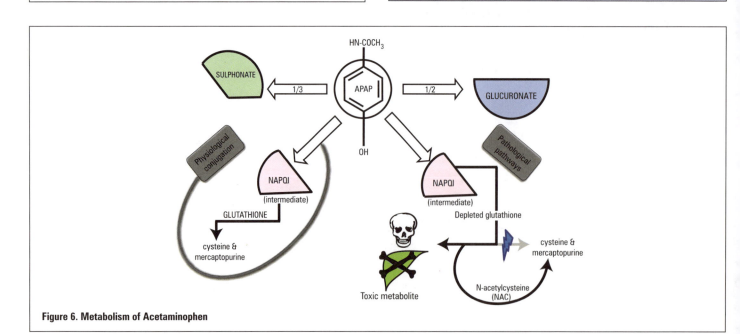

Figure 6. Metabolism of Acetaminophen

Analgesics

Opioids

Also known as narcotics, this class of drug was derived from an extract of the opium poppy *Papaver somniferum*. Opioid is the term used to describe any compound acting at the opioid receptors that has **MORPHINE**-like pharmacological properties. Opiate is the term used to describe naturally occurring alkaloids only (i.e. **MORPHINE** from opium or endogenous opiates such as β-endorphin).

Opioids are classically used for operative and post-operative analgesia and provide better pain control for visceral pain than NSAIDs. Opioid potency and formulations causing euphoria may be highly addictive and dangerous.

Drug	Plasma Half-life (hours)	Activity at Opioid Receptor
Short Half-Life Opioids		
MORPHINE	2-3.5	Agonist
HYDROMORPHONE	2-3	Agonist
OXYCODONE	2-3	Agonist
PENTAZOCINE	2-3	Mixed agonist/antagonist
FENTANYL	3-4	Agonist
CODEINE	3	Agonist (weak)
MEPERIDINE	3-4	Agonist
TRAMADOL	4-6	Agonist
NALOXONE	1-1.5	Antagonist
Long Half-Life Opioids		
METHADONE	24	Mixed agonist/antagonist
BUPRENORPHINE	24-60	Partial Agonist
LOPERAMIDE	9-14	Agonist
NORMEPERIDINE	14-21	Agonist

Opioid Receptors

μ	Mu	Analgesia, miosis, sedation, euphoria, respiratory depression, physical dependence, gastrointestinal dysmotility, bradycardia
κ	Kappa	Analgesia, miosis, diuresis, dysphoria
δ	Delta	Analgesia, modulation of μ-receptor function

Opioid Receptor Distribution in the CNS

1. **Mediating analgesia:** dorsal horn of spinal cord, periaqueductal gray, thalamus
2. **Mediating respiration, cough, nausea and vomiting, pupillary diameter:** ventral brain stem
3. **Affecting neuroendocrine secretions:** hypothalamus
4. **Affecting mood, behaviour, limbic structures:** hippocampus, amygdala, ventral tegmental area, nucleus accumbens

MOA
- Binds to opioid receptors (G-protein coupled receptors)
- Inhibits adenylyl cyclase → activation of inward rectifying K^+ channels, and inhibition of voltage gated Ca^{2+} channels
- Opioid pain modulation:
  - Triggers depolarization of descending pain modulating pathways at the raphe nucleus and periaqueductal gray receptors in brainstem, therefore blocks ascending pathway
- Inhibition at dorsal horn and peripheral terminals of nociceptive afferent neurons
- Opioid activated brain reward pathway:
  - Inhibit GABAergic interneurons → disinhibit ventral tegmental area
- Dopamine independent activity in the nucleus accumbens

USES
- Analgesia
- Sedation
- Anti-diarrhetic (**LOPERAMIDE** and **DIPHENOXYLATE**)
- Anti-tussive (**DEXTROMETHORPHAN** and **CODEINE**)
- Opioid addiction (**METHADONE/BUPRENORPHINE**)

PK
- Metabolized in liver by CYP450

> Differences in **CODEINE** metabolism to **MORPHINE** may be evident due to CYP2D6 polymorphisms → may be clinically relevant.

ADRs
- Respiratory depression
- Bradycardia, hypotension
- QT prolongation (**METHADONE**)
- Seizures (potentially caused by hypoxia due to respiratory depression)
- Acute muscle rigidity (with rapid IV injections of highly potent opioids, i.e. **FENTANYL**)
- Nausea and emesis (via area postrema)
- Miosis (via parasympathetic system)
- Constipation (due to decreased peristalsis)
- Pruritus
- Acute lung injury
- Poikilothermia

> **LOPERAMIDE** is a weak analgesic notable for its constipation side effects → frequently used as anti-diarrhetic in noninfectious cases.

CONTRAINDICATIONS
- Any CNS depressant (i.e. benzodiazepines, alcohol)

Neuroadaptation

TOLERANCE
- Develops as a result of transient or chronic administration
- May require dosage increase
- Often accompanied by physical dependence
- **Is receptor (μ and δ) specific**
  - Receptor phosphorylation interferes with G-protein interaction
  - Receptor internalization through endocytic pathway
- **Develops to specific effects of opioids**
- Analgesia, motor inhibition, sedation
- **Does NOT affect** miosis and respiratory depression

WITHDRAWAL
- Occurs due to compensatory changes in the cell
- **Hyperexcitability** occurs upon removal of opioid agonist
  - Restlessness
  - Extreme anxiety, hostility
  - Vomiting and diarrhea
  - Muscle twitching
  - Hyperphagia
  - Lacrimation, rhinorrhea, and hyperthermia
  - Mydriasis and photophobia
  - Piloerection, or "goose flesh"
  - Dysphoria
  - Cravings
- Can be precipitated almost immediately by opioid receptor antagonist
- Can be abolished by administering more opioid agonist

TREATMENT
- **Overdose treatment = NALOXONE**
  - Opioid receptor competitive antagonist
- **Withdrawal treatment**
  - **METHADONE**
  - **BUPRENORPHINE**
  - **CLONIDINE**

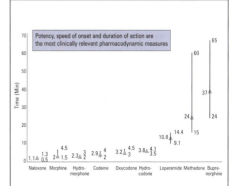

Figure 7. Half-lives of Common Opiates and Antagonists

Benzodiazepines

MOA
- Bind GABA$_A$ receptors between α and γ subunits; increase the frequency of channel opening, enhancing GABA inhibition (requires the presence of GABA)

USES
- First line anxiolytic and sedative-hypnotic agents
- Anxiety
  - Generalized – **DIAZEPAM**
  - Psychotic - **LORAZEPAM**
- Insomnia (hypnosis)
  - Benzodiazepines are closest to ideal hypnotic
  - Suitable only for short term due to compensation
- Epilepsy and seizures
  - More effective against generalized seizures
  - Only used for seizure treatment in short term
    - **MIDAZOLAM**
  - Alcohol and sedative withdrawal – prevent seizures and the intensity of physical withdrawal
    - **CLONAZEPAM, DIAZEPAM**
- Anterograde amnesia
  - Adjunct to decrease presurgical apprehension
  - **MIDAZOLAM**: Colonoscopy, endoscopy
  - **DIAZEPAM**: Laser vision correction
  - **FLUNITRAZEPAM**
    - "Date rape" drug
    - **Class I** controlled substance (NO approved use)
- Muscle relaxation
  - Decrease muscle spasm or pain associated with trauma
  - Cerebral palsy
  - Doses for muscle relaxation lead to excessive sedation
- Alcohol withdrawal
  - Delirium tremens
    - **LORAZEPAM**: Short term
    - **DIAZEPAM**: Long term

PK
- Readily absorbed after oral administration (30 minutes-3 hours)
- CYP450 metabolized → excreted in urine
- **MIDAZOLAM**
  - Highly water soluble, given IM with little pain
  - Very lipid soluble at physiological pH → better sedation → with increased amnestic and anxiolytic effect
- **LORAZEPAM**
  - Fast acting, but short duration
- **DIAZEPAM**
  - Slow onset, but long lasting
  - Short t$_{1/2}$ (4 hours)
  - Metabolized to active metabolites → extended half life
  - **DIAZEPAM → OXAZEPAM** (active)

ADRs
- **Rebound insomnia** (abrupt cessation)
- **Cardiovascular and Respiratory** – very mild effects
  - At high (hypnotic) doses
    - Hypotension and tachycardia
  - Overdose
    - Respiratory depression facilitated if other agents were used concurrently (alcohol, CNS depressants)
  - **MIDAZOLAM** post-op respiratory depression
- CNS
  - CNS depression is dose dependent and potentiated by other depressants
  - Common
    - Drowsy, sedation, hostility, confusion, amnesia, impaired motor coordination
    - At high dose → coma
  - Rare
    - Increased hostility and irritability (like alcohol)
    - Vivid nightmares
- Tolerance and Dependence
  - **Class IV** controlled substance
  - Psychological dependence
  - Gradual withdrawal may avoid some side effects (taper over 10 days-3 weeks)
  - Due to sympathetic over activity
  - Anxiety, delirium, coma, rebound insomnia, hallucinations
  - Benzodiazepine withdrawal shares common features with alcohol withdrawal
  - Progression of events:
    1. Tremor
    2. Myoclonic seizures (aka, grand mal, tonic clonic)
    3. 1 and 2 are repeated with increasing frequency
    4. Status epilepticus (emergency)
    5. Coma
    6. Death
  - Can be alleviated by other sedative-hypnotics
  - Do not use opioids to facilitate withdrawal
  - **ALPRAZOLAM** has high addiction potential
- Paradoxical reactions (~1% of users)

CONTRAINDICATIONS
- Liver disease (short acting benzodiazepines)

NOTES
- Preferred over other anxiolytics (such as barbiturates) because of fewer cardiovascular side effects
- Relatively safe even in overdose

Overdose

FLUMAZENIL
- Benzodiazepine antagonist
- Antagonizes benzodiazepine and **ZOLPIDEM**
- Minimize sedative effect
- Surgical procedures to temporarily wake the patient

Anti-Obesity Drugs

Anti-obesity medications are used in the reduction or maintenance of weight in overweight or obese individuals. Changes in weight can be ascribed to an imbalance of energy input and expenditure. Weight gain occurs when there is energy input in excess of energy expenditure. Input is largely regulated by the gut through absorption and by the CNS via hunger. Expenditure is heavily regulated by an interplay of multiple body systems, including the CNS.

Treatment approaches include decreasing energy input in the gut by decreasing absorption and in the CNS by decreasing appetite. Anti-obesity drugs should only be used when adjustments to diet and activity levels have failed, and even then, should be used in adjunct to these treatments. It should further be noted that comorbid conditions and certain medications may underlie changes in weight, and the use of anti-obesity drugs may not ameliorate the impact of other causes. Consequently, the source of weight gain in a given patient should be understood prior to prescribing these medications.

Other Causes of Weight Gain
- Antipsychotics/steroid hormones: increase energy intake
- β-blockers: decrease energy expenditure
- Decreased glucosuria of diabetes therapy: decrease energy loss
- Endocrine: hypothyroidism, Cushing's syndrome, growth hormone deficiency
- Genetic: Prader-Willi syndrome, Bardet-Biedl syndrome

ORLISTAT
MOA
- Inhibits gastric and pancreatic lipases
  - Avoids hydrolysis of triglycerides in gut
  - Fats are excreted undigested
  - Results in steatorrhea and frequent bowel movements

USES
- Modest weight loss

PK
- Short $t_{1/2}$ (1-2 hours)

ADRs
- Malabsorption of vitamins A, D, E, K
- Hepatotoxicity (rare)
- Acute renal impairment (rare)

CONTRAINDICATIONS
- Chronic malabsorption syndrome

DRUG INTERACTIONS
- CYCLOSPORINE
- AMIODARONE

PHENTERMINE
MOA
- Stimulates release of NE to enhance satiety
- Sympathomimetic

USES
- Appetite suppressant in obese patients

PK
- Long $t_{1/2}$ (~20 hours)

ADRs
- Cardiovascular effects (hypertension, tachycardia, arrhythmias)
- Dry mouth
- Nervousness and anxiety
- Insomnia

CONTRAINDICATIONS
- Hyperthyroidism
- Hypertension

DRUG INTERACTIONS
- MAO inhibitors

NOTES
- PHENTERMINE is a controlled substance

Antipsychotics

Antipsychotics (Neuroleptics)

Antipsychotics target dopamine (DA) neurotransmission, particularly within the mesocortical dopamine pathway. Specifically, antipsychotics are D_2 receptor antagonists and reduce dopamine neurotransmission in the brain. At the appropriate doses, all antipsychotics have the same therapeutic efficacy, although finding the appropriate drug for a particular patient usually involves trial and error. Response to antipsychotics begins in the first week of treatment and accumulates over time. One major challenge in the treatment of psychotic patients is compliance. Suicide rates are high among patients with schizophrenia, but the antipsychotic medications are relatively safe in overdose, and are therefore not a major concern in this context. Antipsychotics are not addictive, but tolerance may develop; withdrawal after high-dose treatment may reveal latent dyskinesias.

Classes of Antipsychotics

Typical Antipsychotics (CHLOROPROMAZINE, FLUPHENAZINE, HALOPERIDOL)
- These drugs are associated with adverse effects caused by dopamine receptor antagonism (e.g. extrapyramidal motor symptoms, galactorrhea, etc.)

Atypical Antipsychotics (CLOZAPINE, OLANZAPINE, ARIPIPRAZOLE, QUETIAPINE, RISPERIDONE)
- These drugs are often associated with weight gain, hyperlipidemia and type 2 diabetes as adverse drug reactions

Common Properties of Antipsychotic Drugs

TARGET DOPAMINE NEUROTRANSMISSION
- Psychotic behaviors are linked to overactive dopamine neurotransmission, specifically the **mesocortical** pathway
  - Major pathways utilizing dopaminergic transmission:
    - Tuberoinfundibular pathway
    - Mesolimbic pathway
    - Nigrostriatal pathway
    - Mesocortical pathway

CONTRAINDICATIONS
- Drugs which activate dopaminergic pathways (these drugs would exacerbate psychotic behaviors)
  - Amphetamine (triggers DA release)
  - Levodopa (increases DA activity, replenishes DA stores)
  - Cocaine (inhibits DA reuptake, thereby prolonging its action)

PK
- Highly lipid soluble and thus cross the blood brain barrier
- **Large volume of distribution**

ADRs
- More common with typical antipsychotics
- Elevation in prolactin: due to inhibition of DA signaling along the tuberoinfundibular pathway
- **Movement disorders:** extrapyramidal signs (EPS) due to inhibition of DA signaling along the nigrostriatal pathway; mnemonic – TRAPS
  - **T**remor
  - Muscle **R**igidity
  - **A**kinesia
  - Stooped **P**osture
  - **S**huffling Gait

BINDING TO OTHER RECEPTORS
- Typical and atypical antipsychotics bind to other receptors, including 5-HT and ACh receptors, and can result in adverse reactions from this non-specific binding

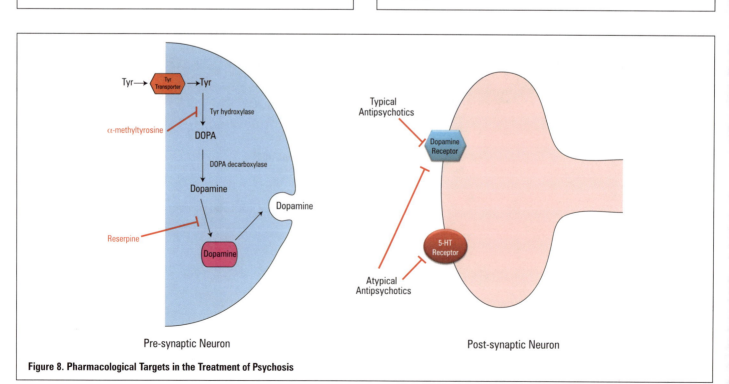

Figure 8. Pharmacological Targets in the Treatment of Psychosis

Antipsychotics

Typical Antipsychotics

Phenthiazines	Butyrophenones
CHLORPROMAZINE	FLUPHENAZINE
	HALOPERIDOL

MOA
- Blockade of D_2 receptor

USES
- Psychosis
- Schizophrenia
- Acute mania
- Tourette syndrome

PK
- **CHLORPROMAZINE:** Short $t_{1/2}$ (~6 hours)
- **FLUPHENAZINE, HALOPERIDOL:** Very long $t_{1/2}$ (10-38 hours)

ADRs
- Anticholinergic effect (BLUSH PADS BBC) (see Autonomic Drugs chapter)
- Sedation
- Endocrine side effects (due to disinhibition of prolactin release, thus resulting in increased gonadotropin release)
  - Galactorrhea
  - Gynecomastia
  - Inhibition of ovulation
  - Amenorrhea
- Vasodilation (due to α_1 receptor blockade)
  - Sexual dysfunction
  - Orthostatic hypotension
  - Syncope
  - Reflex tachycardia
- Cholestatic jaundice
- Hypersensitivity reactions
  - Agranulocytosis, photosensitivity, urticaria, contact dermatitis
- Interference with temperature regulation
  - Usually hyperthermia, sometimes hypothermia

EXTRAPYRAMIDAL (EPS) EFFECTS
- **Acute Dystonia**
  - Spasms of muscles of face, tongue, and neck
  - Treated using anti-muscarinics and anti-histamines
- **Akinesia**
- **Akathisia**
  - Strong subjective feelings of distress or discomfort
  - Treated by reducing dose or by switching drugs
- **Tardive Dyskinesia**
  - Lip smacking, choreiform limb movements
    - May be irreversible (avoided by using lowest doses of drug)
- **Pseudoparkinsonism**
  - Ridigity, tremor, shuffling gait
    - Develops over period of days to weeks
    - Due to striatal D_2 receptor blockade
    - Treated using anti-parkinsonian drugs
- **Neuroleptic Malignant Syndrome**
  - **Rare life-threatening disorder** that resembles parkinsonism with hyperthermia
    - 10% mortality
  - Days to weeks progression
  - Risk can be minimized by gradual dose escalation
  - Treatment: immediately stop neuroleptic, plus supportive care. **DANTROLENE** and **BROMOCRIPTINE** may be helpful, but antiparkinsonian drugs are not helpful

Atypical Antipsychotics

MOA
- Blockade of D_2 receptor
- Target several receptors (not specific to the DA receptor)
- Advantage: targets positive and negative symptoms
- Negative symptoms include affect flattening, alogia, and avolition

USES
- Psychosis
- Schizophrenia
- Antiemesis
- Decreasing alcoholic hallucinations
- Treatment of intractable hiccup
- Treatment of extreme agitation

ADRs
- Weight gain and/or Type 2 diabetes

CLOZAPINE
PK
- Moderate $t_{1/2}$ (8-12 hours)

ADRs
- Lowers seizure threshold (at high doses)
- Agranulocytosis (risk highest during beginning of therapy)
- Hypersalivation

CONTRAINDICATIONS
- Epilepsy
- Agranulocytosis

NOTES
- Very few extrapyramidal effects and no prolactin release

OLANZAPINE
USES
- Schizophrenia
- Bipolar disorder
- Anxiety disorders
- Treatment-resistant depression

PK
- Very long $t_{1/2}$ (21-54 hours)

ADRs
- Dyslipidemia

ARIPIPRAZOLE
USES
- Bipolar disorder
- Major depressive disorder
- Autism

PK
- Very long $t_{1/2}$ (~75 hours)

QUETIAPINE
USES
- Schizophrenia
- Bipolar disorder
- Major depressive disorder

PK
- Short $t_{1/2}$ (6 hours)

ADRs
- Sedation
- Orthostatic hypotension

RISPERIDONE
USES
- Schizophrenia
- Bipolar disorder

PK
- Long $t_{1/2}$ (20-30 hours)

ADRs
- Increased risk for excess prolactin release

Mood Disorders

Major Depressive Disorder and Bipolar Disorder (Manic-Depressive Disorder)

Depressive disorders are typically characterized by episodes of depressed mood and/or anhedonia that last at least 2 weeks. These periods often include disturbances in sleeping patterns, changes in appetite, and may involve thoughts of death and suicide. Traditionally, MAOIs and TCAs have been used to treat depressive episodes. More recently, SSRIs and SSNRIs have become the first line of therapy. Though the mechanism by which these agents exert antidepressant effects remains unknown, the proximal effects are on neurotransmitter function. The "monoamine hypothesis" suggests that alterations in serotonin, noradrenaline, and dopamine may be involved in mood disorders. Consequently, medications that modulate neurotransmitter levels can help reduce depressive symptoms in these patients.

Bipolar disorder can include depressive episodes, but is mainly characterized by manic episodes lasting at least one week. These involve prolonged states of elevated mood, along with feelings of grandiosity, hyperactivity, and reduced need for sleep. Lithium is the prototypical mood stabilizer, though antiepileptic drugs or atypical antipsychotics are also commonly used to treat manic episodes.

The antidepressants have a therapeutic lag and require at least 2-3 weeks (or longer, up to 6 weeks) to work. This lag time may be due to the role of neurogenesis in mediating the effects of antidepressant drugs. Typically, when treating a newly diagnosed patient, one would start with an SSRI and titrate an adequate dose.

If complete remission is not attained, one would first choose another SSRI. In the case that SSRIs do not work, a TCA should be tried. MAOIs are used as a last resort. Major depression that is refractory to all drug treatment may be treated using electroconvulsive therapy. Treatment with antidepressants may precipitate manic episodes in bipolar patients.

It is important to note that antidepressant drugs can have fatal interactions when used together. When switching between classes of antidepressants, at least 2 weeks should be allowed to avoid serious drug interactions. The potential for overdose must be considered. Depressed patients are at risk for suicide and therefore care must be taken when using drugs with narrow therapeutic windows for the treatment of depression. Drugs with low therapeutic indices include the TCAs and the MAOIs. SSRIs, on the other hand, have very wide therapeutic windows and are, therefore, safer in overdose. Eating disorders frequently co-exist with mood disorders, therefore antidepressants may be useful for these patients. Caution must be taken, however, to adjust dosage to the patient's lean body mass.

All antidepressants have a black box warning for use in children and adolescents. This is NOT a contraindication. Rather, it is more of a warning of increased risk of suicide. The risk of suicide should be weighed against the benefits; pediatric patients on antidepressants must be carefully monitored for this reason.

Treatment Options for Major Depressive Disorder

Selective serotonin reuptake inhibitors (SSRIs) and Selective serotonin-norepinephrine reuptake inhibitors (SSNRIs)

Tricyclic antidepressants (TCAs)

Monoamine oxidase inhibitors (MAOIs)

Other drugs affecting monoamine neurotransmitters

Treatment Options for Bipolar Disorder

Lithium

Antiepileptic drugs

Atypical antipsychotic drugs

Selective Serotonin Reuptake Inhibitors (SSRIs)

FLUOXETINE, PAROXETINE, SERTRALINE, CITALOPRAM

MOA
- Highly specific inhibitor of 5-HT reuptake

USES
- First line treatment for depression
- Anxiety disorders (panic disorder, obsessive-compulsive disorder, PTSD)
- Eating disorders
- Premenstrual dysphoric disorder

PK
- Long $t_{1/2}$ (1-3 days)
  - Metabolites may have very long $t_{1/2}$ (norfluoxetine; 4-16 days)

ADRs
- Nausea, anxiety, nervousness, headache
- Sexual dysfunction
- Changes in appetite/weight
- Risk of suicidal ideation (greatest during first few months of therapy)
- Cardiovascular effects, including EKG changes (very rare)

CONTRAINDICATIONS
- Liver impairment

DRUG INTERACTIONS
- MAOIs (may cause serotonin syndrome)

Selective Serotonin-Norepinephrine Reuptake Inhibitors (SSNRIs)

VENLAFAXINE, DULOXETINE

MOA
- Inhibitor of 5-HT and NE reuptake (5-HT > NE)

USES
- Similar to SSRIs
- Neuropathic pain (**DULOXETINE**)

PK
- Moderate $t_{1/2}$ (5-12 hours)

ADRs
- Similar to SSRIs
- Sweating

CONTRAINDICATIONS
- Liver impairment
- Closed angle glaucoma (**DULOXETINE**)

DRUG INTERACTIONS
- MAOIs

Mood Disorders – Antidepressants

Tricyclic Antidepressants (TCAs)

IMIPRAMINE, AMITRIPTYLINE

MOA
- Block 5-HT and NE reuptake

USES
- Depression
- Panic disorders
- Urinary incontinence
- Noctural enuresis
- ADHD
- Neuralgia or fibromyalgia

PK
- **IMIPRAMINE**
  - Moderate to long $t_{1/2}$ (6-18 hours)
- **AMITRIPTYLINE**
  - Moderate to long $t_{1/2}$ (9-25 hours)

ADRs
- Antimuscarinic effects (dry mouth, urinary retention, constipation)
- Cardiovascular effects (orthostatic hypotension, tachycardia, hypertension, arrhythmias, T-wave abnormalities)
  - Dose-dependent cardiotoxicity
- CNS effects (sedation, decreased seizure threshold, delirium, confusion)

CONTRAINDICATIONS
- Seizure disorders

DRUG INTERACTIONS
- MAOIs (may cause hypertensive crisis and hyperpyrexia)
- Drugs that prolong QT interval
- Alcohol (may potentiate CNS depression)

Monoamine Oxidase Inhibitors (MAOIs)

PHENELZINE, TRANYLCYPROMINE

MOA
- Non-selectively and irreversibly inhibits all MAOs
  - Increases concentration of 5-HT, DA, and NE
- MAO-A: ubiquitous, MAO-B: brain-specific

USES
- Third line of treatment for depression (after SSRIs and TCAs)
- Atypical (refractory) depression
- Anxiety and panic disorder
- Hypochondria

PK
- **PHENELZINE**
  - Long $t_{1/2}$ (~12 hours)
- **TRANYLCYPROMINE**
  - Shor $t_{1/2}$ (2-4 hours)

ADRs
- CNS stimulation
- Insomnia
- Agitation or hypomania (common)
- Seizure, confusion, or hallucination (rare)

CONTRAINDICATIONS
- Cardiovascular disease
- Cerebrovascular disease

DRUG INTERACTIONS
- Substances containing or affecting levels of catecholamines
  - TCAs, tyramine-containing foods
- SSRIs (such as **FLUOXETINE, PAROXETINE**) or tryptophan ("serotonin syndrome")

Other Drugs Affecting Monoamine Neurotransmitters

MAPROTILINE

MOA
- Strong inhibition of NE reuptake, weak inhibition of 5-HT reuptake
- Moderate anti-histaminergic and anti-cholinergic activity

PK
- Very long $t_{1/2}$ (30-60 hours)

ADRs
- Anti-cholinergic effects
- Strong sedation at beginning of therapy
- Seizures

CONTRAINDICATIONS
- Epilepsy

DRUG INTERACTIONS
- MAOIs

TRAZODONE

MOA
- Serotonin antagonist and reuptake inhibitor

PK
- Moderate $t_{1/2}$ (~7 hours)

ADRs
- Sedation
- Nausea
- Dizziness
- Headache
- Blurred vision
- Priapism

BUPROPION

MOA
- Inhibits reuptake of NE and DA

USES
- Smoking cessation

PK
- Long $t_{1/2}$ (1 day)

ADRs
- Seizure (especially in the context of eating disorders)
- Stimulant effects (agitation, insomnia, tremor)
- Nausea, dry mouth, sweating

CONTRAINDICATIONS
- Epilepsy
- Bulimia and/or anorexia

DRUG INTERACTIONS
- MAOIs
- Inducers/inhibitors of CYP2B6
- Abrupt discontinuation of alcohol or sedatives may increase risk for seizures

Mood Disorders – Mania

LITHIUM

LITHIUM

MOA
- Currently unknown but thought to stabilize receptor activity by interfering with the phosphatidylinositol pathway:
  - Inhibits the hydrolysis of inositol, thus reducing the release of intracellular second messengers, IP_3 and DAG, in the brain
- Other possible effects on neurotransmission and cation transport

USES
- Treatment and prophylaxis of mania or manic depressive (bipolar) disorder
- May be used in combination with
  - Antipsychotics or benzodiazepines; for severe mania
  - Antidepressants; for manic depressive disorder

PK
- Excreted in urine
- Long $t_{1/2}$ (24 hours)
- $t_{1/2}$ increases with continuous therapy

ADRs
(Often due to alterations in Na^+ transport in nerve cells, muscle cells, and in the renal tubule)
- CNS effects (confusion, tremors, aphasia, motor hyperactivity)
- Gastrointestinal disturbances
- CV effects (arrhythmias, hypotension, edema)
- Renal effects (polyuria, polydipsia (nephrogenic diabetes insipidus))
- Hypothyroidism
- Long term therapy may cause renal damage

CONTRAINDICATIONS
- Renal impairment (drug monitoring recommended)
- Significant cardiovascular disease
- Sodium-restricted diet
- Severe dehydration

DRUG INTERACTIONS
- NSAIDS, diuretics, ACE inhibitors; elevate serum levels by reducing Li^+ clearance

NOTES
- Narrow therapeutic window
  - Therapeutic drug monitoring for lithium blood levels is required (normal range is 0.5 to 1.3 mM, >1.5 mM is toxic)
- Delayed onset (up to 2-3 weeks)
  - Can co-administer with mood stabilizers initially

Antiepileptics and Antipsychotics for Mixed Manic States (Simultaneous Depression and Mania)

CARBAMAZEPINE

MOA
- Centrally acting ion channel blocker

USES
- Epilepsy
- Symptomatic relief of trigeminal neuralgia
- Alone or in combination with Li^+ for the treatment of mania and prophylaxis of manic depressive disorder

PK
- Hepatic metabolism
- Excreted in urine
- Long $t_{1/2}$ (25-65 hours for a single dose)
- Due to autoinduction of enzymes, the $t_{1/2}$ after repeated doses is 12-17 hours

ADRs
- CNS effects (drowsiness, confusion, dizziness, ataxia)
- Visual disturbances (diplopia, blurred vision, nystagmus)
- Nausea/vomiting

CONTRAINDICATIONS
- History of or present bone marrow depression

DRUG INTERACTIONS
- Many drug interactions due to CYP450-inducing properties
- May cause agranulocytosis and not to be used with **CLOZAPINE**
- Concomitant use of MAOI, or during 2 weeks of discontinuing an MAOI
- Concomitant use of **NEFAZODONE** may reduce drug efficacy

NOTES
- Delayed onset
- Narrow therapeutic window
- Close clinical and frequent laboratory supervision should be maintained throughout treatment
- Smallest dose is sufficient for antimanic effects
- **See Antiepileptics**

VALPROATE ACID

MOA
- Acts as an indirect GABA agonist by inhibiting GABA transaminase
- Use dependent ion channel blocker

USES
- Seizures
- Alone or in combination with Li^+ for manic depressive disorder
- Migraine prophylaxis

PK
- Hepatic metabolism
- Excreted in urine
- Long $t_{1/2}$ (9-16 hours)

ADRs
- Nausea/vomiting
- Weight gain
- Tremors

CONTRAINDICATIONS
- Hepatic impairment
- Urea cycle disorders

DRUG INTERACTIONS
- Inhibits the metabolism of **PHENOBARBITAL**, **PHENYTOIN**, and **CARBAMAZEPINE**
- Some drug interactions due to CYP450-inducing properties

NOTES
- Therapeutic drug monitoring required for **VALPROATE ACID**

OLANZAPINE (atypical antipsychotics)

MOA
- Unknown, thought to be mediated through combination of dopamine and serotonin antagonism

USES
- Schizophrenia and related psychotic disorders
- Manic or mixed episodes associated with manic depressive disorder

PK
- Hepatic metabolism
- Very long $t_{1/2}$ (21-54 hours)

ADRs
- Drowsiness
- Weight gain, increased appetite
- Hyperglycemia/hyperlipidemia
- Orthostatic hypotension
- Xerostomia (dry mouth)
- Sedation

DRUG INTERACTIONS
- Increased risk of cardiotoxicity with concurrent use of **LEVOMETHADYL**

Anxiolytics and Sedative-Hypnotics

Sleep

- **Non-REM sleep**
  - Stage 1 – Light sleep, desynchronous EEG
  - Stage 2 – Deepening sleep, increasingly synchronous
  - Stage 3 – Deepening sleep, increasingly synchronous
  - Stage 4 – Deep sleep, synchronous
- **REM sleep**
  - Period of heightened brain activity, rapid eye movement, and muscle relaxation where dreaming occurs
    - EEG resembles that of the wakeful state
- Neurotransmitters that mediate sleep
  - GABA
    - Projections from the ventrolateral preoptic nucleus (VLPO in hypothalamus) to the reticular activating system (RAS)
    - Inhibits activity of the RAS, the wake center, and promotes sleep

Wakefulness

Wakefulness is set by a balance of excitation and inhibition mediated by the reticular activating system (RAS)
- Neurotransmitters that mediate wakefulness
  - Acetylcholine
    - Projections from the basal forebrain to the entire cerebral cortex
    - Additional projections from the mesopontine to the thalamus (enhance excitatory glutamatergic transmission to the cerebral cortex)
  - Norepinephrine
    - Projections from the locus ceruleus (upper pons) to the cerebral cortex
  - Serotonin
    - Projections from the raphe nuclei to the entire forebrain.
  - Dopamine
    - Projections from the VTA of the midbrain to limbic and cortical structures
  - Histamine
    - Projections from interneurons in the tuberomammillary nucleus of the hypothalamus, to broad areas of the brain

NOTES
- Serotonergic and noradrenergic projections inhibit mesopontine cholinergic neurons important for muscle atonia characteristic of REM sleep

DEFINITIONS
- **Tranquilizer**
  - An agent that reduces mental disturbances (tension, anxiety), and promotes calmness
- **Sedative**
  - An agent that decreases activity, agitation, and calms the patient while having little effect on motor or mental function
- **Hypnotic**
  - An agent that induces drowsiness and promotes and maintains sleep
  - Generally patients can be easily aroused by external stimuli
- **General Anesthesia**
  - An agent that induces unconsciousness and decreases ones response to stimuli
  - Patients are not easily aroused, even by intense stimuli

Anxiolytics

MOA
- Promote inhibition in the amygdala via $GABA_A$
- Decrease sympathetic activation especially adrenergic (locus ceruleus)
- Block serotonin receptors (raphe nuclei)

Sedative-Hypnotics

WITHDRAWAL
- Physical dependence may develop and manifest as withdrawal symptoms following discontinuation of the drug
  - **I**nsomnia
  - **A**NS hyperactivity (tachycardia, sweating, tachypnea, etc.)
  - **T**remor
  - **S**eizures
  - **H**allucinations
  - **D**elirium
- Symptoms may be confused with original symptoms prevailing before onset of drug
- Some can be life-threatening thus, to minimize symptoms, patients must be titrated slowly off the drugs by gradually tapering the dose.

> *Important **A**lways **T**aper **S**edative-**H**ypnotic **D**oses.*

- Severity of the syndrome depends on drug pharmacokinetics
- Mild withdrawal:
  - Long-acting drugs whose prolonged elimination allows time for receptors to return to normal state
- Severe withdrawal:
  - The rapid elimination of short-acting drugs does not allow enough time for receptors to return to normal

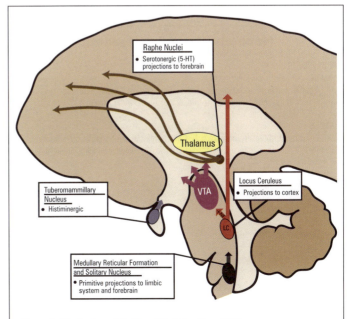

Figure 9. Mechanism of Action of Sedative-Hypnotics

Anxiolytics and Sedative-Hypnotics

Barbiturates

SECOBARBITAL, THIOPENTAL, BUTABARBITAL, PHENOBARBITAL

MOA
- Increases the duration of channel opening and enhances affinity for GABA by binding the beta subunit of the $GABA_A$ receptor chloride channel
- Barbiturates can activate the GABA chloride channel without the presence of GABA
- Inhibit excitatory AMPA receptors at synapse

USES
- Sleep, pre-operative sedation
- Anticonvulsant
- Anesthetic

PK
- Primary difference between barbiturates is their duration of action
- Ultra-short acting (**THIOPENTAL**)
  - Very lipid soluble → enters CNS rapidly
  - Anesthetics (20 minutes)
- Short/Intermediate acting (**SECOBARBITAL**)
  - Moderate lipid soluble → enters CNS slower
  - Longer duration of action
- Long acting (**APROBARBITAL, PHENOBARBITAL**)
  - Low lipid solubility
  - Slow onset (1 hour), long duration (6-12 hours)

ADRs
- Coughing, sneezing, laryngospasm, hiccoughing
- Drowsiness, confusion, mood distortion, hangover, hypersensitivity (localized swelling), nausea, vomiting, diarrhea
- Paradoxical excitement
- High dependence potential
- Overdose → CNS and PNS depression, depressed respiration and CV system, coma, death

NOTES
- Potentiates other CNS depressants
- VERY dangerous to mix with alcohol
- Induction of CYP450
- Adverse drug reactions worse than benzodiazepines and thus replaced by benzodiazepines

Nonbenzodiazepine Hypnotic

ZOLPIDEM

MOA
- Agonist for a subset of the benzodiazepine site on $GABA_A$ receptor
- Not in the same class as benzodiazepines, but similar MOA

USES
- Sedation without anticonvulsant, muscle relaxation or significant amnesia
- Sleep – decreased latency, increased time, little effect on sleep cycle

PK
- Rapid absorption and quick onset
- Short $t_{1/2}$ (3 hours)

ADRs
- Drowsiness, dizziness, ataxia
- Diarrhea
- Dependence – Class IV

NOTES
- No morning hangover

Atypical Sedative-Hypnotics

BUSPIRONE

MOA
- Partial agonist of serotonin receptor

USES
- Chronic treatment of anxiety

PK
- Short $t_{1/2}$ (2 hours)

ADRs
- Tachycardia, palpitations, GI distress, dizziness

NOTES
- Lower potential for dependence
- 1-2 week therapeutic lag
- Advantage: does not potentiate other CNS depressants

CHLORAL HYDRATE (chloral derivative)

MOA
- Unknown, but results from the active metabolite, trichloroethanol

USES
- Insomnia
- Sedation
- Alcohol withdrawal syndrome

PK
- Moderate $t_{1/2}$ (4-12 hours)

ADRs
- Nausea, vomiting
- Hallucinations

Over-the-Counter (OTC) Sleep Aids

DIPHENHYDRAMINE, DOXYLAMINE, HYDROXYZINE PAMOATE
- H_1 histamine antagonists
- Sedative-hypnotics
- Sedation → anxiolytic properties
- Do not produce consistently effective sleep
- Included in most OTC sleep aids
- Tolerance develops
- Potential for overdose

Sympatholytics

PROPRANOLOL

MOA
- Antagonizes β-adrenergic receptors
- Blocks the adrenergic response associated with anxiety

USES
- Anxiety, panic attacks

NOTES
- See Cardiovascular Drugs chapter

CLONIDINE

MOA
- Agonizes $α_2$-adrenergic receptors of locus ceruleus
- Stimulates negative feedback circuits to decrease release of norepinephrine

USES
- Anxiety → stops tachycardia, mydriasis, sweating
- Less effective for blocking emotional component of anxiety

NOTES
- See Antipsychotics section

Drugs of Abuse

Mesolimbic Reward Pathway

For there to be abuse potential, a drug must elicit the reward pathway to compel positive feelings and addiction.

The **mesolimbic pathway** is the central pathway within the pleasure and reward circuit. This **predominantly dopaminergic** pathway can be modulated by different drugs of abuse to cause feelings of pleasure.

<u>Hallucinogens</u> (LSD, mescaline, psilocybin, etc.) are not active in the reward pathway, and therefore <u>not addictive</u>.

This circuit relates to reward and is not necessarily responsible for the intoxicating effects of each drug. The following common effects, however, can be associated with imbalances in monoamine neurotransmitters:
- **NOREPINEPHRINE (NE)** → tachycardia, hypertension, vasoconstriction, diaphoresis, tremor, pupillary dilation (mydriasis)
- **DOPAMINE (DA)** → anorexia, stereotyped movements, hyperactivity, sexual excitement

TERMINOLOGY
- **Addiction** → A recurring compulsion by an individual to engage in activities, despite harmful consequences; tolerance and physiological dependence are not hallmarks of addiction in the same manner as psychological dependency
- **Physical Dependence** → An abnormal physiologic state brought about by repeated administration of a drug that manifests as withdrawal symptoms when the drug is stopped or decreased
- **Psychological Dependence** → Craving and compulsive use of a drug to produce pleasure or avoid discomfort despite negative effects on health and personal life
- **Tolerance** → Decreased sensitivity to a drug, and its effects, that develops as a result of repetitive exposure thus necessitating subsequently larger doses to achieve desired effects
- **Cross-Tolerance** → Exposure to one substance produces tolerance to another

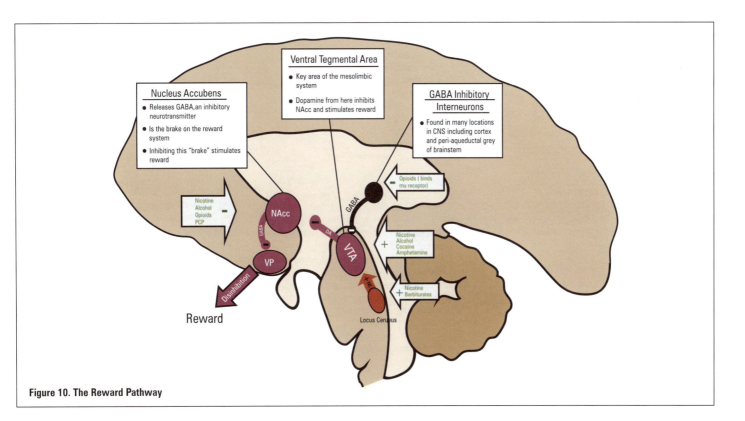

Figure 10. The Reward Pathway

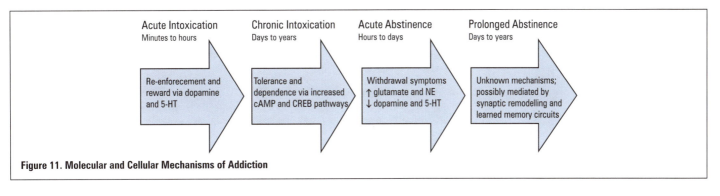

Figure 11. Molecular and Cellular Mechanisms of Addiction

Drugs of Abuse – Stimulants

MOA
- Effects of psychostimulants result from **monoamine reuptake block**:
  - **NE** → tachycardia, hypertension, vasocontriction, diaphoresis, tremor, pupillary dilation (mydriasis)
  - **DA** → anorexia, stereotyped movements, hyperactivity, sexual excitement, stereotypy, paranoia, hallucinations
  - **5HT** → euphoria, hyperthermia

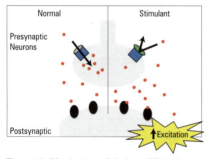

Figure 12. Mechanism of Action of Stimulants

USES
- Treatment of ADHD
- Obesity
- Narcolepsy
- Treatment resistant depression (rarely)

INTOXICATION	WITHDRAWAL
CNS Stimulation	**CNS Depression**
• Euphoria	• Dysphoria
• Agitation	• Strong cravings
• Hypervigilance	
• Hyperthermia	
• Impaired judgment	
• Seizures	
Psychomotor Agitation	**Psychomotor Retardation**
• Stereotyped behaviors	
• Hyperreflexia	
• Dyskinesia	
• Stereotypy	
• Dystonia	
Increased Energy	**Fatigue**
• Decreased sleep	• Increased sleep
Anorexia	**Hyperphagia**
Autonomic Arousal	
• Tachycardia	
• Tremor	
• Mydriasis	
• Diaphoresis	
Cardiorespiratory Irregularity	
• Dysrhythmia	
• Chest pain	
• Respiratory depression	
• Hypertension	
• Vasospasm/Constriction	
• Tachypnea	
• Myocardial infarction	
• Stroke	

ECSTACY/MDMA = 3,4 - Methylenedioxy methamphetamine
("E", "X", candy, e-bomb, love drug)
- May contain other amphetamine derivatives such as MDA and MDEA in addition to MDMA
- Entactogenic amphetamine

MOA
- Increase release of DA and NE, block reuptake of 5-HT
- Affects mainly **5-HT** neurons originating in the raphe nuclei
  - Raphe nuclei project and blanket the cortex
  - Serotonin released all at once, **and** inhibits reuptake → floods the cortex
- Serotonin flood → leads to neurotoxicity
  - DA depletion → **motor dysfunction**

PK
- Moderate $t_{1/2}$ (7.5 hours)
- Metabolized by CYP2D6

ADRs
- **Hyperthermia** is the greatest short term risk
  - Coagulation (disseminated intravascular coagulopathy)
  - Rhabdomyolysis
  - Seizures
- Bruxism
- **Neurotoxicity**
  - Depression
  - Memory deficits
  - Impaired mental function

COCAINE
(coke, crack, blow, yeyo, base, kryptonite)

MOA
- Blocks reuptake of 5HT>NE>DA into the presynaptic cell
- **DA** build up at synapse → **strong addiction** due to reward circuit activation
- At high dose → blocks voltage gated Na⁺ channels, inhibiting neurotransmission thus acting as a **local anesthetic**

USES
- Increased energy, alertness, confidence and euphoria

PK
- Short $t_{1/2}$ (60 minutes)
- Metabolized in plasma and liver → urine (detectable up to 3 days)

ADRs
- Overdose usually results in cardiotoxicity, dysrhythmia and extreme hypertension (powerful vasoconstrictor), tachycardia, tachypnea, hyperthermia
- Withdrawal symptoms are depressive (see table)
- Mydriasis
- Obstetrical issues: abruptio placentae

AMPHETAMINES
(speed, crank, meth, ice, Ritalin®)

MOA
- Taken up into cell by reuptake pumps (especially DA pumps)
- Disrupt vesicular storage of monoamines:
  - Monoamines rise in concentration in the cytosol
  - Monoamines are pumped out by reversal of the reuptake pump

USES
- Delayed onset of mental/physical fatigue

PK
- Long $t_{1/2}$ (~7-30 hours)

ADRs
- Extensions of excessive sympathomimetic stimulation:
  - Hypertension
  - Hyperpyrexia
  - Severe tachycardia and collapse
  - Delirium
  - Convulsions

NOTES
AMPHETAMINE and **DEXTROMETHAMPHETAMINE**
- Abuse of prescription ADD and ADHD medication

METHAMPHETAMINE
- More potent than amphetamine
- Is the drug of choice of abusers

Amphetamine Syndrome
- May occur at high doses of amphetamines
- Gives rise to acute psychotic picture, including:
  - Hyperactivity
  - Paranoia/Delusions
  - Auditory/Tactile hallucinations
  - Patient maintains clear consciousness and no disorientation

Drugs of Abuse – Opioids

Opiates
(China white, chasing the dragon, junk, horse, smack, percs, killer, O.C., oxy, etc.)

MECHANISM OF ACTION
- Opioids bind to opioid receptors
  - Mu, delta, kappa G protein coupled receptors
  - Inhibit adenylate cyclase
    - **Activate** inward rectifying K^+ channels
    - **Inhibit** voltage gated Ca^{2+} channels
  - Ultimately reduce excitability and transmitter release of neurons
- Two mechanisms for opioid activated brain reward
  - Disinhibit VTA by inhibiting GABAergic interneurons
  - DA independent activity in the NAcc

PK
- Metabolized in liver → urine excretion

> **Opioids** refer to any chemical (natural or synthetic) that binds to the opioid receptors. **Opiates** refer to the natural alkaloids derived from the opium plant (e.g. **MORPHINE, CODEINE**)

Neuroadaptation
- Chronic use → loss in desired properties, with gain of reinforcing properties
- Tolerance is receptor specific
  - Mu couples less well to G proteins during chronic treatment
- Tolerance develops to specific effects of opioids:
  - Analgesia and motor inhibition
  - Depressant properties
- Tolerance does NOT occur with:
  - Miosis
  - Respiratory depression
  and therefore are diagnostic and important signs to look for

- Factors that yield abuse:
  - **Reinforcing** effects work by relieving:
    - **Dysphoria** = restlessness and dissatisfaction
    - **Withdrawal** symptoms
  - **Intense craving**

INTOXICATION	WITHDRAWAL
Stimulation • Experience a rush early on • Sedation and apathy after initial phase Note: may cause dysphoria in some	**Depression** • Dysphoria • Anxiety and hostility • Cravings
Sensations of Warmth & Flushing • Whole body itching caused by histamine release	**Piloerection** • Aka 'goose flesh', lacrimation, rhinnorhea and hyperthermia
Analgesia	**Hyperphagia**
Constipation	**Diarrhea** • Cramping, nausea, vomiting
Miosis (pin point pupils)	**Mydriasis and Photophobia**
Respiratory Depression • Apnea/cyanosis • Hypotension • Nausea and vomiting	**Yawning** • Tachypnea

Treatment
- The most commonly abused opiates include
  - **HEROIN**
  - **MORPHINE**
  - Prescription opiates (**OXYCODONE**)

- Treat <u>overdose</u> with opiate antagonist (**NALAXONE**)

- Treat <u>withdrawal</u> symptoms with **METHADONE/BUPRENORPHINE** (± **CLONIDINE**)

OPIOID SUBSTITUTION THERAPY
- Long term corrective therapy for opioid dependence
- Aims to reduce withdrawal symptoms and drug cravings, while improving health and lifestyle
- Pharmacological treatment in combination with psychosocial support is most effective
  - **METHADONE** Maintenance Therapy
  - **BUPRENORPHINE**, alone or in combination with **NALOXONE** (SUBOXONE)
    - **NALOXONE** has poor oral absorption, but reduces potential for **BUPRENORPHINE** abuse

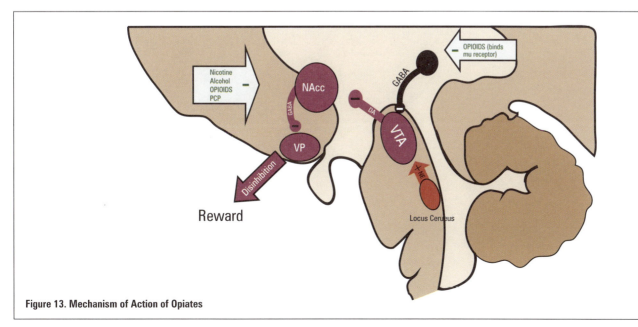

Figure 13. Mechanism of Action of Opiates

Drugs of Abuse – Nicotine

MOA
- Binds to **nicotinic acetylcholine receptor (nAChR)** centrally to enhance DA release in the reward pathway, and peripherally to stimulate both the sympathetic and parasympathetic nervous systems. Nicotinic receptors are Na^+/K^+ channels that depolarize neurons or muscle end plates; effects include:
  - NMJ – stimulates end plate depolarization
  - Autonomic ganglionic – stimulates both sympathetic and parasympathetic nervous systems causing hypertension, tachycardia, coronary artery constriction, arrhythmia, tremor, nausea, vomiting, diarrhea, dyspepsia, etc.
  - Adrenal medulla – stimulates release of epinephrine and NE
  - Centrally
    - VTA, striatum, Nacc, SNpc and cortex
    - Causing lightheadedness, alertness, anorexia and insomnia

PK
- Inhaled **NICOTINE**:
  - Avoids 1st pass metabolism
  - Reaches brain in 7 to 10 secs post-inhalation (provides rapid onset)
- Oral **NICOTINE** (chewing **TOBACCO**; capsule)
  - 1st pass metabolism
- Mainly hepatic metabolism
- Renal clearance (5-35%)
- Short $t_{1/2}$ (2-4 hours)

INTOXICATION – Is not a DSM IV diagnosis

DRUG SEEKING
- **Craving** – especially after eating or during stress; but variable from person to person

INTOXICATION	WITHDRAWAL
Stimulation	Depression
• Increased alertness	• Difficulty concentrating
• Mild euphoria	• Irritability and craving
Muscle Relaxation	Restlessness and Anxiety
Nausea and Anorexia	Increased Appetite
Increased Psychomotor Activity	Hyperventilation

Therapy

NICOTINE REPLACEMENT THERAPY
- Many patches, gums and inhalers exist and each has its own adverse reaction and efficacy profile
- Different methods of administration (nicotine gum, nicotine inhaler, nicotine lozenge, nicotine nasal spray, nicotine patch)

USES
- **NICOTINE** cessation
- Advantage – delivers **NICOTINE** without toxins and carcinogens present in tobacco smoke

PK
- Slow release – administer nicotine more slowly than via cigarettes

1. SHORT ACTING PRODUCTS
NICOTINE GUMS/SPRAY/INHALER/LOZENGES
- Releases nicotine into the bloodstream over 20-30 minutes
- Absorption of 1 mg of **NICOTINE** (via gum) is approximately equal to <1-3 mg of **NICOTINE** absorbed (via smoking)
- Steady state plasma concentrations achieved with chewing **NICOTINE** gum hourly is **much lower** than **NICOTINE** concentrations with smoking

2. LONG ACTING PRODUCTS
NICOTINE PATCH
- **NICOTINE** levels in the blood rise over hours
- Releases **NICOTINE** in an even manner, reducing the risk of peak and trough nicotine concentrations in bloodstream over 20-30 minutes
- Patch users receive 50% less **NICOTINE** compared to smokers

NOTES
- Adjust dose based on symptoms
- Combinations of nicotine replacement products may be used

BUPROPION
MOA
- Inhibits reuptake of NE and DA
- May block nACh-receptors

USES
- Smoking cessation
- Depression

NOTES
- See Antidepressants section

VARENICLINE
MOA
- nAChR partial agonist

USES
- Smoking cessation with 12 weeks of therapy
  - If successful with cessation – additional 12 weeks therapy to further increase the likelihood of long term smoking cessation

ADRs
- Suicidal ideation
- Nausea
- Insomnia
- Mood change

> Despite therapy almost 90% of users relapse!

Neuroadaptation
- **Dependence** is indicated by difficulty quitting
- Reinforcing
- **Down regulated DA receptors**
- **Upregulated nAChR** due to temporary nAChR inactivation by nicotine shortly after binding and activating it

CHRONIC USE EFFECTS
- COPD
- Clotting problems
- Different forms of cancer
- Cardiovascular effects

NOTES
- Psychiatric co-morbidities very common among smokers:
  - Schizophrenia patients (70-88% are smokers)
  - Depression
  - ADHD (40% are smokers)
- PREGNANCY: Adverse pregnancy outcome associated with **NICOTINE** use in pregnancy: growth restriction, preterm deliveries, spontaneous abortion, stillbirth
- LACTATION: **NICOTINE** found in breast milk at concentrations approximately twice those found in blood

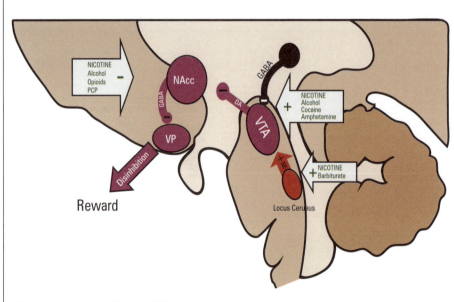

Figure 14. Mechanism of Action of Nicotine

Drugs of Abuse – Cannabinoids and Hallucinogens

Cannabinoids
(Weed, ganja, pot, bud, reefer, mary jane, joint, blunt, cheeba, dope, etc.)

Principal active ingredient – **THC (DELTA-9-TETRAHYDROCANNABINOL)**
Concentration of **THC** varies across three most common types of **CANNABINOIDS**:
1. **MARIJUANA** (1-14% **THC**) – most commonly used illicit drug in US
2. **HASHISH** (2-8% **THC**)
3. **HASH OIL** (highly potent 15-50% **THC**)

ANANDAMIDE is an endocannabinoid (a naturally occurring cannabinoid in the body)

MOA
- Bind to and activate CB_1 receptors (CB = **C**anna **B**inoid), to produce psychoactive effects, and CB_2 receptors
- CB_1 is a G protein coupled receptor
  - Found throughout the forebrain
  - Receptor locations and cannabinoid effects
    - Basal ganglia → locomotor activity
    - Cerebellum → coordination
    - Hippocampus → memory
    - Hypothalamus → regulate food intake
  - Inhibit adenylate cyclase and Ca^{2+} mediated neurotransmitter release
- **THC** induces DA release in the NAcc (like **NICOTINE**)
- **THC** increases activity of DA neurons in the VTA

USES
- Prevention of chemotherapy-induced emesis
- Appetite stimulation
- Glaucoma, multiple sclerosis, epilepsy, anxiety
- Chronic pain management
- Recreational drug
- Routes of administration
  - Smoking (provides rapid onset intense "high")
  - Oral – via food

EARLY INTOXICATION (~1-30 minutes)	LATE EFFECTS (~1-3 hours)
Euphoria	Sedation
• Uncontrollable laughter	• Continued euphoria
	• Irritability and craving
Psychoactive Effects	
• Anxiety, paranoia	
Hallucinations and Dissociations	
• Sensations of slowed time • Auditory and visual distortions	
Increased Appetite	
• The "munchies" and xerostomia (dry mouth)	
Tachycardia	
Conjunctival Reddening	
• Reddening of the eyes and ptosis/squinting of the eyelids	

PK
- Very lipophilic
- It may take several weeks for THC to be cleared (up to 4 weeks)
- Metabolized in liver to another psychoactive compound
  - **11-HYDROXY-THC**

ADRs
- Psychosis
- Shortened attention span
- Poor judgment
- Impaired communication skills
- Diminished effectiveness in interpersonal situations

NOTES
- **Tolerance** develops with increased use
- No DSM IV classified withdrawal

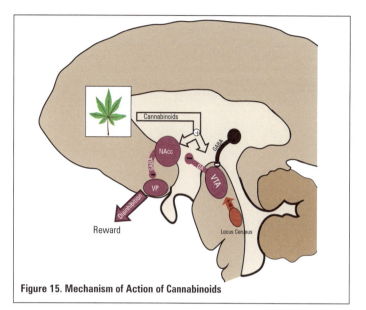

Figure 15. Mechanism of Action of Cannabinoids

Hallucinogens

LYSERGIC ACID DIETHYLAMINE (LSD), PSILOCYBIN, MESCALINE

MOA
- Act primarily at 5-HT receptors (not $5-HT_3$ or $5-HT_4$)
  - Hallucinogenic effects mediated via $5-HT_{2A}$
- Also activates DA receptors and adrenoreceptors

USES
- Abused for hallucinogenic properties
- Tested as experimental treatment for cluster headaches, psychotherapy

PK
- **LSD:** Short $t_{1/2}$ (3-4 hours)
- **PSILOCYBIN:** Short $t_{1/2}$ (~1 hour)
- **MESCALINE:** Short $t_{1/2}$ (~6 hours)

ADRs
- Autonomic arousal (tachycardia, palpitations)
- Tremors and incoordination
- Psychological reactions during episode
  - May exacerbate pre-existing psychiatric illness
- Hallucinogen Persisting Perception Disorder (HPPD)
  - "Flashbacks", often visual disturbances, that occur while not under influence of drug

NOTES
- Tolerance quickly develops when taken at short intervals
  - Due to rapid down-regulation of $5-HT_2$ receptors
  - Cross-tolerance common between hallucinogens
- No withdrawal effects or dependence develop

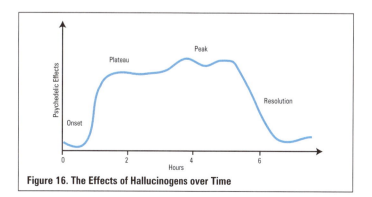

Figure 16. The Effects of Hallucinogens over Time

Drugs of Abuse – Dissociative Anesthetics

Though initially developed as anesthetics, dissociative anesthetics have been frequently abused for the hallucinogenic effects that they produce. These compounds are differentiated from other hallucinogens by the feelings of detachment, or dissociation, from the self. Individuals under the influence of these drugs are often not ambulatory, and have a distorted or lost sense of time.

PHENCYCLIDINE (PCP)
MOA
- Non-competitive antagonists of Ca^{2+} channels on NMDA receptors
  - Cortex and hippocampus → cognitive impairments
- Activation of DA neurons in VTA
- Stimulate release and inhibit reuptake of NE
  - Causes disrupted motor activity

PK
- Very long $t_{1/2}$, but highly variable (7-50 hours)
- Liver hydroxylation → kidney excretion
- Inhibits CYP2C11 and CYP2D activity

ADRs
- Sympathomimetic effects (tachycardia, hypertension, hyperthermia)
- Muscle rigidity
- Seizures
- "PCP coma" (may last up to 2 weeks)
  - Prolonged period of psychotic behaviour
- Schizophrenia-like psychosis

Effects of Dissociative Anesthetics

Low Doses
- Analgesia
- Emotional withdrawal
- Stereotypy
- Euphoria
- Excitement and agitation

Moderate Doses
- Anesthesia
- Catatonic posturing
- Hallucinations
- Aggressive behaviour
- Amnesia

High Doses
- Loss of ego
- Loss of sense of time
- Psychotic episodes
- Long-lasting amnesia
- Stupor or coma

KETAMINE
MOA
- Non-competitive antagonists of Ca^{2+} channels on NMDA receptors
  - Cortex and hippocampus → cognitive impairments
- Activation of DA neurons in VTA
- Binds μ and Σ opioid receptors

USES
- Used as anesthetic in human and veterinary medicine
- Considered a date rape drug

PK
- Short $t_{1/2}$ (2-3 hours)
- Two phases:
  - α ($t_{1/2}$ = ~15 minutes), corresponds with anesthetic effects
  - β ($t_{1/2}$ = ~2.5 hours)

ADRs
- Depression of respiratory reflex
- Nausea
- Cognitive and memory impairments (after chronic use)
- Delirium and amnesia
- Impaired motor function

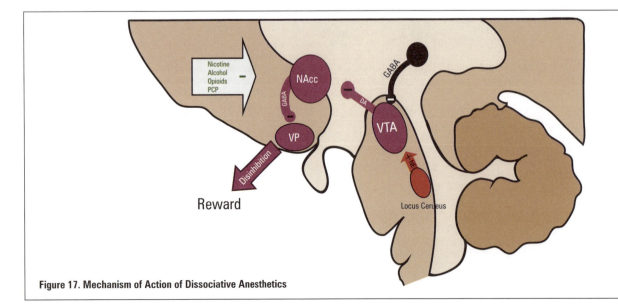

Figure 17. Mechanism of Action of Dissociative Anesthetics

Drugs of Abuse – Depressants and Volatile Inhalants

Depressants

A diverse group of drugs that decrease CNS and motor activity and include alcohol, GHB and sedative-hypnotics.

GHB

GAMMA HYDROXY BUTYRATE (GHB)
- Produced naturally by body in small amounts
- **CNS depressant** → relaxation and relief from anxiety
  - Reduced inhibitions
- **Enhances the depressant mechanisms of alcohol and benzodiazepines**
- Higher doses can depress vital functions such as breathing leading to deep sleep, coma or death
- Intoxicating effects begin with 10 minutes; lasts up to 4 hours
  - Often used in **date rape** sexual assaults
- Addictive and with chronic users → prolonged withdrawal (months)

INTOXICATION	WITHDRAWAL
Disinhibition • Inappropriate sexual or aggressive behavior • Impaired judgment and mood swings • Impaired attention and memory	**Agitation** • Anxiety • Psychomotor agitation • Sensory distortions (visual, auditory and tactile) and hallucinations
Somnolence	**Tremor and Insomnia** • Delirium and seizures
Incoordination • Unsteady gait • Nystagmus	**Autonomic Hyperactivity** • Tachycardia, sweating, hypertension

Sedatives/Hypnotics and Anxiolytics

CLINICAL USES
- Insomnia
- Anxiety
- Seizure disorders
- Muscle relaxants
- Significant withdrawal

BENZODIAZEPINES (BZD)
FLUNITRAZEPAM = **date rape** drug
- Severe withdrawal in people with tolerance
  - **Delirium tremens** → **seizures**
- BZD's require GABA to be present to have any effect

MOA AND EFFECTS
- In a drug **naïve patient**, yields acute effects:
  - Open the ionotropic $GABA_A$ chloride channel maximally only when GABA is also present
  - Enhanced inhibitory neurotransmission → causing anxiolytic actions

- However, in a **chronic user/abuser**, tolerance and dependence leads to
  - Adaptive changes GABA-R causing the chloride channel to open less than before but still enough to give an anxiolytic or euphoric effects
  - Excessive actions of BZDs at the same receptor that mediate the therapeutic actions are thought to be the psychopharmacological mechanism of euphoria, drug reinforcement, and overdose

- **Acute withdrawal** in a BZD dependent individual
  - **Dysphoria, headache and depression** instead of euphoria
  - **Anxiety and agitation** instead of tranquility
  - **Insomnia** instead of sedation and sleep
  - **Muscle tension** instead of muscle relaxation
  - **Convulsions** instead of anticonvulsant effects
  - Weight loss and **paresthesias**

BARBITURATES
- Can open the GABA chloride channel **independent of GABA binding**

Volatile Inhalants

- **Anesthetics** – nitrous oxide
- **Industrial and household solvents** – paint thinners, solvents in glues, correction fluid, markers, pen solvents
- **Gases and aerosols** – butane lighters, aerosol cream dispensers, spray paint, hair spray
- **Aliphatic nitrites** – amyl nitrite (poppers)

NITROUS OXIDE, AMYL NITRATE
MOA
- Inhibiting activity of NMDA receptors
- Body becomes starved for oxygen → heart rate picks up

PK
- Inhaled vapors readily absorbed into the circulatory system
- High lipophilicity results in rapid access to the brain
- **Lungs are important route of excretion**
- Single "sniff" does not cause long-lasting CNS effects
- **Rapid and short acting** → can be used more than once per hour

ADRs

ORGAN	DAMAGE CAUSED BY INHALANT
Blood and marrow	Decreased O_2 carrying capacity; leukemia
Heart	Sudden Sniffing Syndrome (SSS) caused by fatal arrhythmia
Skin	'Glue sniffers' rash around nose and mouth; runny nose
CNS	CNS hypoxia with resultant memory loss, slurring of speech, deafness, uncoordination, personality changes and hallucinations
PNS and muscle	Paresthesias, paralysis and muscle wasting

Drugs of Abuse – Alcohol

Ethyl alcohol (ethanol) is the psychoactive component responsible for alcohol's effects. Having minimal therapeutic use, it has become the most ubiquitous drug used and a serious public health issue.

MOA
- Not well understood, but thought to interact through several mechanisms
  - Direct membrane effects
    - Readily diffuses into lipid membranes affecting the fluidity and function of membrane associated proteins such as receptors and ion channels
  - Receptor mediated effects
    - Increases GABA-receptor mediated inhibition
    - Inhibits glutamate NMDA-receptor activation thus, reducing excitation
      - May have important role in learned alcohol consumption behavior and memory of euphoria
    - Potentiates serotonin activity at $5\text{-}HT_3$ receptors, which are localized on inhibitory interneurons → enhancing inhibition
    - Release of dopamine into the nucleus accumbens → euphoria

USES
- Antidote for methanol poisoning

PK
- Rapidly absorbed from the stomach (20%) and small intestine (80%)
- Absorption rate is dependent on concentration
- The presence of food delays gastric emptying and alcohol absorption
- Distributes into total body water and across the blood brain barrier
- Hepatic metabolism follows zero-order kinetics; metabolism is independent of concentration
- On average, an adult can metabolize 1 drink of alcohol/hour

- Primary pathway for metabolism is via alcohol dehydrogenase (ADH), which is saturated at high alcohol concentrations
- Ethanol can induce and be metabolized by CYP2E1
  - In heavy drinkers, 20% of alcohol intake is metabolized by CYP2E1
- Polymorphisms exist for ADH and acetaldehyde dehydrogenase (ALDH) and are common in people of Asian descent and influence risk of alcohol dependency
- Acetaldehyde is responsible for unpleasant side effects; facial flushing, nausea, vomiting, dizziness, and headache
- Most ethanol is completely oxidized to CO_2 and H_2O
- 2-10% of consumed alcohol is excreted by the lungs, in the urine and sweat

NOTES
- Binge drinking refers to 5 (males) or 4 (females) or more standard drinks on one occassion (generally within 2 hours)
- Heavy drinking refers to 2 (males) or 1 (females) per day

Effects

Acute use: CNS and cardiovascular effects
Chronic use: Systemic effects

CENTRAL NERVOUS SYSTEM
- **Acute Effects:** State of "Intoxication"
  - Sedation
  - Euphoria
  - Slurred speech
  - Ataxia
  - Mood swings
  - At lethal concentrations of blood ethanol, can induce coma, respiratory depression, or death
  - Amounts of alcohol for the manifestation of this state is dependent on the individuals tolerance
    - Chronic alcoholics may be conscious with a BAC of 0.4 % or more
- **Chronic Effects**
  - Cerebral atrophy
  - Memory loss
  - Alcoholic psychosis
  - Peripheral nerve injury
  - Impaired visual acuity
  - Sleep disturbances
    - Reduces latency and causes sleep fragmentations
  - If deficient in thiamine, may lead to Wernicke-Korsakoff syndrome
    - Paralysis of external eye muscles, ataxia, and confusion

- Chronic consumption of large quantities of alcohol can result in tolerance and dependence
  - **Tolerance:** can occur at the metabolic or cellular level
  - **Withdrawal:** results in a stimulation of the CNS
    - Result from upregulation of glutamate receptors during chronic alcohol use, so in withdrawal have hyperactivity
  - **Psychological Dependence:** most important factor leading to alcoholism

CARDIOVASCULAR SYSTEM
- **Acute Effects**
  - Systemic vasodilation
- **Chronic Effects**
  - Cardiomyopathy
  - Hypertension
  - Arrhythmias

LIVER
- **Chronic Effects**
  - Promotes the development of fatty liver → alcoholic hepatitis → cirrhosis → liver failure

GASTROINTESTINAL SYSTEM
- **Chronic Effects**
  - Denatured enzymes
  - Increased gastric secretions
  - Gastric mucosal inflammation and irritation, which can lead to erosive gastritis
    - Exacerbates gastric damage induced by aspirin
  - Increased pancreatic secretion and duct obstruction may lead to chronic pancreatitis
  - May cause diarrhea, constipation, weight loss, and vitamin deficiencies

OTHER EFFECTS
- **Endocrine/Metabolic Effects**
  - Altered fluid/electrolyte levels
  - Hypoglycemia and ketosis
- **Renal Effects**
  - Inhibition of antidiuretic hormone causes increased urination
  - Decreased tubular water reabsorption
- **Increased risk of cancers**

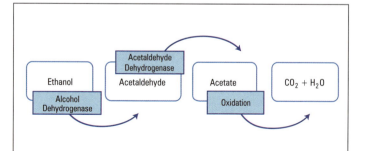

Figure 18. Metabolism of Ethanol

Drugs of Abuse – Alcohol Abuse and Dependence

DRUG INTERACTIONS
- Due to CYP450-inducing properties, may increase or inhibit the metabolism of other drugs
- Chronic use increases susceptibility to acetaminophen hepatotoxicity
- Potentiates the effects of
  - Sedative-hypnotics
  - Vasodilators
  - Oral hypoglycemic agents
- Cross-tolerance exists with alcohol and sedative-hypnotics and general anesthetics

PREGNANCY
- Consumption of alcohol in pregnancy can lead to fetal alcohol spectrum disorder (FASD)

WITHDRAWAL SYNDROME
- Symptoms develop around 6-8 hours after alcohol consumption is stopped
- Minor withdrawal (48-72 hours)
  - Anxiety
  - Insomnia
  - Tremor
  - Hypertension
  - Sweating
  - Nausea and vomiting
- Severe withdrawal
  - Visual hallucinations
  - Tonic-clonic seizures
  - Disorientation
  - Arrhythmias
  - Delirium tremens (can be fatal if not treated)

SCREENING TOOLS
- Screening tools for identification of patients at risk for alcohol abuse are available (i.e. CAGE questionnaire)

Blood Alcohol Concentration (BAC)
- Often used as a measure of intoxication
- Expressed as a percentage of volume of alcohol per volume of blood in the body
- Is affected by: gender, body weight, time spent drinking, gastric contents
- Legal limits range from ~0.05-0.08%
- Lethal BAC ~0.40% and greater
- Estimating BAC
  - $BAC = 0.02*(n-t)$
  - n = oz. of 80 proof alcohol, or the number of 12 oz. beers
  - t = number of hours since consumption
  - Assuming a 70 kg person with normal liver function
- Example: A 25 year old college student weighing 225 lbs. consumes eight 12 oz, 6% alcoholic beverages in two hours. His BAC at three hours (after he began drinking) would be: $(8 - 3) \times (0.02) \times (70/100) = 0.10 \times 0.7 = 0.07\%$

Management and Treatment

MINOR WITHDRAWAL
- Restore potassium, magnesium, and phosphate imbalances only if renal function is normal
- Thiamine and vitamin B_{12} – for the prevention of Wernicke-Korsakoff syndrome

SEVERE WITHDRAWAL
- BENZODIAZEPINES are the DOC for treating the symptoms of alcohol withdrawal
- Begin with a large dose, then gradually taper the dose, based on PK and symptoms, over several days (adjust dose based on the Clinical Institute Withdrawal Assessment (CIWA) scale score)
- **DIAZEPAM** (see *Benzodiazepines*)
- **LORAZEPAM** (see *Benzodiazepines*)

ACUTE ALCOHOL INTOXICATION (Overdose)
- Supportive Care
  - Maintain airway and support respiration to prevent respiratory depression and aspiration of vomitus
  - If unconscious, try to rouse and immediately seek medical attention
- Medical Care
  - IV fluids with thiamine, multivitamins and magnesium
  - Glucose may be administered if metabolic imbalances exist
    - May potentiate phosphate imbalances – monitor serum levels
  - Differential diagnosis – screen for other drugs or other cause for coma

ALCOHOLISM
- Drug therapy and counseling, in combination, is useful in treating alcohol associated conditions and to prevent relapse

NALTREXONE (see *Opioids*)
MOA
- Opioid antagonist, competitive binding at receptors

USES
- Dosed daily to decrease cravings and maintain abstinence

PK
- Hepatic metabolism
- Excreted in urine
- Very long $t_{1/2}$ (5-10 days)

ADRs
- Gastrointestinal disturbances
- Headache

CONTRAINDICATIONS
- Severe hepatic impairment
- Physical dependence on opioids

DRUG INTERACTIONS
- Opioids and opioid containing products
- Concurrent use with **DISULFIRAM** should be avoided – both are potential hepatotoxins

ACAMPROSATE
MOA
- Weak NMDA-receptor antagonist and $GABA_A$-receptor activator → stabilizes neurotransmitter imbalances associated with alcohol dependency

USES
- Dosed three times/day to reduce cravings and maintain abstinence

PK
- Poor absorption which is reduced by food
- Excreted in urine
- Long $t_{1/2}$ (20-33 hours)

ADRs
- Gastric disturbances

CONTRAINDICATIONS
- Renal impairment: a dose adjustment is necessary

DISULFIRAM
MOA
- Irreversibly binds ALDH
- Results in the accumulation of acetaldehyde which is responsible for the unpleasant reaction to alcohol
  - **Acetaldehyde syndrome**: flushing, nausea, headache, vomiting, dizziness, sweating, hypotension, and confusion

USES
- Dosed daily for the
  - Maintenance of alcohol abstinence
  - Treatment of chronic alcoholism
- Should only be used if patient has abstained from alcohol for at least 12 hours

PK
- Hepatic metabolism
- Very long $t_{1/2}$ (days)

ADRs
- Dermatitis
- Garlic-like or metallic aftertaste
- Hepatotoxicity

CONTRAINDICATIONS
- Coronary occlusion
- Relative psychoses
- Severe myocardial disease

DRUG INTERACTIONS
- Concurrent use of ethanol and ethanol-containing products (mouthwashes, cough syrups, etc.)
- Concomitant use of **PARALDEHYDE**, **METRONIDAZOLE**, and **AMPRENAVIR** may potentiate toxic effects
- Some drug interactions due to CYP450-inhibiting properties
- **PHENYTOIN, CHLORDIAZEPOXIDE, BARBITURATES, WARFARIN**

NOTES
- Diethyldithiocarbamate is a toxic metabolite that is an effective chelator of copper and other metals
- Inhibits the activity of metalloenzymes such as; dopamine beta-hydroxylase, alcohol dehydrogenase

Endocrine Drugs

Chapter Authors: Andrew W. Browne, Jennifer Galle and Jennifer A. O'Malley

Faculty Reviewers: I. George Fantus and Bernard P. Schimmer

IN THIS CHAPTER

Thyroid 106
    Hypothyroidism
    Hyperthyroidism

Antidiabetic Drugs 109
    Type 1
    Type 2

Corticosteroids 112

DRUGS IN THIS CHAPTER

Generic Name	US Trade Name	Canadian Trade Name
acarbose	PRECOSE	GLUCOBAY
aminoglutethimide	CYTADREN	
betamethasone	CELESTONE	BETAJECT, CELESTONE, SOLUSPAN
dexamethasone	DECADRON, DEXPAK, MAXIDEX, OZURDEX	DEXASONE, MAXIDEX
fludrocortisone	FLORINEF	
glyburide	DIABETA, MICRONASE	DIABETA
hydrocortisone	ANUSOL, AQUANIL, CETACORT, COLOCORT	CORTEF, CORTENEMA, CORTODERM, HYCORT, PREVEX, SARNA
insulin aspart	NOVOLOG	NOVORAPID
insulin determir	LEVEMIR	
insulin glargine	LANTUS	
insulin lispro	HUMALOG	
ipodate	ORAGRAFIN, GASTROGRAFIN	
ketoconazole	NIZORAL, XOLEGEL, EXTINA	KETODERM, NIZORAL
levothyroxine	LEVOTHYROID, LEVOXYL, SYNTHROID, UNITHROID, TIROSINT	ELTROXIN, EUTHYROX, SYNTHROID
liothyronine	CYTOMEL, TRIOSTAT	CYTOMEL
liotrix	THYROLAR	
metformin	FORTAMET, GLUCOPHAGE, RIOMET, GLUMETZA	GLUCOPHAGE, GLUMETZA
methimazole	TAPAZOLE	
metyrapone	METOPIRONE	
perchlorate		
pioglitazone	ACTOS	
prednisone	DELTASONE, PREDNICOT, STERAPRED	DIOPRED, PRED FORTE, PRED MILD
propranolol	INDERAL, INNOPRAN	INDERAL
propylthiouracil		PROPYL-THYRACIL
repaglinide	PRANDIN	GLUCONORM
rosiglitazone	AVANDIA	
spironolactone	ALDACTONE	

Thyroid

Function of Thyroid Hormones

- Maintain proper development and differentiation of all cells of the human body
- Regulate basal metabolic rate (BMR) by regulating metabolism of carbohydrates, lipids, protein, vitamins
  - Calorigenesis and thermogenesis resulting from regulation of numerous rate-limiting steps of metabolism.
- Regulate synthesis, secretion, degradation, and function of hormones such as catecholamines, corticosteroids, antidiuretic hormones, estrogen, and insulin

Thyroid Hormone and Synthesis and Release

Thyroxine (T_4) and Tri-iodothyronine (T_3)
- Synthesized in the thyroid from tyrosine and iodine
  - Note: main source of iodine is dietary intake
- Synthesis of T_3 and T_4
  1. Active transport of iodide into follicular cells (**iodide trapping**)
  2. Thyroid peroxidase carries out two reactions:
     a. Iodination: iodide is oxidised to iodine; iodine is then incorporated into tyrosine residues bound (by a peptide linkage) to thyroglobulin (TG) forming mono- or di-iodinated tyrosine (MIT and DIT)
     b. Condensation: iodinated tyrosine residues are then converted to iodo-thyronines, T_4 and T_3
  4. **Thyroglobulin-bound T_3 and T_4** is stored in the follicle lumen as colloid
  5. Endocytosis of thyroglobulin-bound T_3 and T_4 with subsequent lysosomal fusion
  6. **Proteolysis of TG** produces free T_4 and T_3, which exits the cell and enter the circulation
  7. More than 99% of T_3 and T_4 are bound to thyroxin binding globulin (TBG) in the circulation
  8. A small fraction of circulating hormone is free (unbound) and biologically active
  9. **T_4 is converted to T_3 in peripheral tissues by thyroid deiodinase (5'-DID)**

Regulation of Thyroid Hormone Synthesis

Thyroid Stimulating Hormone (TSH)
- Synthesized in the anterior pituitary
- Regulation of TSH synthesis
  - Stimulated by hypothalamic TSH releasing hormone (TRH)
  - Inhibited by circulating T_4, intrapituitary T_3, somatostatin
- TSH regulates:
  - Iodine uptake
  - TH synthesis
- TSH regulates both processes by binding to two receptors (based on the concentration of circulating TSH) on thyroid follicular cells:
  - Ganglioside receptor (signals via cAMP)
  - Glycoprotein receptor (signals via IP_3 and DAG)

Mechanism of Action of Thyroxine (T_4) and Tri-iodothyronine (T_3)

- TH receptors are found in the entire body except spleen and testes
- Thyroid hormone in peripheral tissue binds to a nuclear thyroid hormone receptor (TR) which modulates transcription and protein expression. Expression of TH-responsive genes is stimulated while other genes are repressed. The net effect is cell remodelling in response to TH stimulation
- Affinity of TR for T_3 is ~10-fold higher than T_4
  - All significant action is by T_3
- High levels of thyroid hormone and resultant over-expression of proteins in peripheral tissues causes clinical symptoms of hyperthyroidism

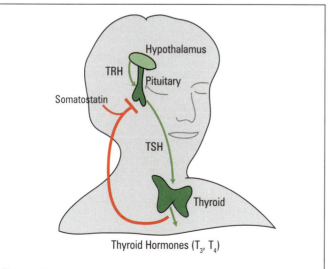

Figure 1. Hypothalamic-pituitary-thyroid Axis

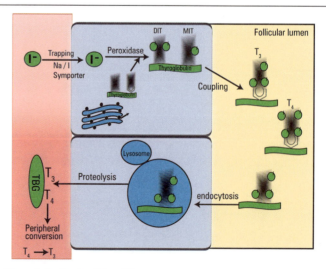

Figure 2. Synthesis of T_3 and T_4

Thyroid – Hypothyroidism

CAUSES
- **1° Hypothyroidism**
  - Thyroid hypothyroidism → TH deficiency
  - Many causes
    - Iatrogenic: post-ablative (I^{131} or surgical thyroidectomy)
    - Autoimmune: Hashimoto's thyroiditis (most common)
    - Hypothyroid phase of subacute thyroiditis
    - Infiltrative disease (progressive systemic sclerosis, amyloid)
    - Iodine deficiency
    - Congenital (1/4,000 births); if untreated: short stature, mental retardation, large tongue, distended abdomen
  - Drugs
    - **AMIODARONE** (anti-arrhythmic drug)
    - **LITHIUM** (for bipolar disorder)
    - **NITROPRUSSIDE** (anti-angina drug)
- **2° Hypothyroidism**
  - Pituitary hypothyroidism → TSH Deficiency
- **3° Hypothyroidism**
  - Hypothalamic hypothyroidism → TRH deficiency

CLINICAL PRESENTATION
- General: fatigue, cold intolerance, slowing of mental and physical performance, enlarged tongue
- CVS: bradycardia, generalized atherosclerosis, pericardial effusion
- GI: anorexia, weight gain, constipation
- Neuro: paresthesia, slow speech, muscle cramps, hung reflexes
- GU: menorrhagia, ammenorrhea, anovulatory cycles
- Derm: puffiness of face, periorbital edema, cool, dry and rough skin, dry and course hair, thinned eyebrows (lateral 1/3)
- Heme: anemia (pallor)

Medical Emergency: Myxedema coma (hypothyroidism, stupor, hypoventilation, hypothermia, bradycardia, hypertension)

DIAGNOSIS
- Based on thyroid function test (blood test)
  - **1° hypothyroidism (TH deficiency)** → most common (90%)
    - Characterized by:
      - Elevated serum TSH levels
      - Decreased serum total T_4 levels (i.e. free and bound) and free T_3 levels
    - Hashimoto's Thyroiditis: Antibodies present against peroxidase and thyroglobulin
  - **2° hypothyroidism (TSH deficiency)**
    - Characterized by low levels of serum TSH that does not increase following TRH (thyrotropin) administration
  - **3° hypothyroidism (TRH deficiency)**
    - Characterized by low levels of serum TSH that increases upon TRH (thyrotropin) administration

Treatment of Hypothyroidsim

- **Therapeutic goal is to normalize thyroid hormone level and prevent myxedema and myxedema coma without causing hyperthyroidism**
- Treatment of hypothyroidism is straightforward: thyroid hormone replacement

ADVERSE REACTIONS
- Most common: hyperthyroidism (due to drug overdose)

LEVOTHRYOXINE

USE
- Outpatient

CONTENT
- Pure synthetic T_4

EFFECTS ON HORMONE LEVELS
- Normal thyroid function tests

ADVANTAGES/DISADVANTAGES
- Slow onset of action - must be converted to T_3
- Very long $t_{1/2}$ (5-7 days)
- Conversion to T_3 by 5'-DID gives tissue some control over T_4 activity
- Drug interactions common

LIOTRIX

USE
- Outpatient

CONTENT
- T_4 and T_3 mixture (4:1)

EFFECTS ON HORMONE LEVELS
- Normal thyroid function tests

ADVANTAGES/DISADVANTAGES
- Both short-acting and long-acting effects
- Mimics natural hormone secretion
- No advantage over **LEVOTHYROXINE**

LIOTHYRONINE

USE
- Inpatient (e.g. myxedema coma)

CONTENT
- Pure synthetic T_3

EFFECTS ON HORMONE LEVELS
- Low serum T_4
- Normal to high T_3
- Normal TSH

ADVANTAGES/DISADVANTAGES
- Fast onset of action
- Very long $t_{1/2}$ (1 day)
- Requires twice daily dosing
- High T_3 toxicity (T_3 is 10x more active than T_4)
  - Hyperthyroidism

Thyroid – Hyperthyroidism

CAUSES
- Graves' Disease
  - B-lymphocytes produce antibodies, directed against TSH receptors that mediate thyroid stimulation (thyroid-stimulating immunoglobulins, TSI)
  - These lymphocytes are not susceptible to negative feedback, leading to an increase in thyroid hormone concentration in blood → thyrotoxicosis
- Toxic multi-nodular goiter
- Toxic nodule
- Thyroiditis

CLINICAL PRESENTATION
- General: fatigue, heat intolerance, irritability, fine tremor
- CVS: tachycardia, atrial fibrillation, palpitations
- GI: weight loss with increased appetite, thirst, hyperdefecation
- Neuro: proximal muscle weakness
- GU: scant menses, decreased fertility
- Derm: fine hair, skin moist and warm, vitiligo, soft nails with onycholysis
- MSK (rare): decreased bone mass, hypercalcemia
- Heme: leukopenia, lymphocytosis, splenomegaly, lymphadenopathy

Medical Emergency: Thyroid storm (severe state of uncontrolled hyperthyroidism, extreme fever, tachycardia, vomiting, diarrhea, vascular collapse and confusion)

DIAGNOSIS
Based on thyroid function test (blood test)

Disorder	TSH	T_4/T_3	Thyroid Antibodies	RAIU*
Graves' Disease	↓	↑	TSI	↑
Toxic multi-nodular Goiter	↓	↑	–	↑
Toxic Nodule	↓	↑	–	↑
Thyroiditis				
• Classical subacute thyroiditis			+/–	
• Silent thyroiditis			–	
• Post partum thyroiditis	↓	↑	+/–	↓

* Radioactive iodide uptake

IODINE SUPPLEMENT
- Increases trapping but INHIBITS organification
- Temporarily effective (1 week); eventually will exacerbate hyperthyroidism
- Degranulates mast cells → allergic-like response

IPODATE (Contrast media)
- Increases trapping but INHIBITS organification
- No adverse reactions directly from IPODATE → adverse effects occur when iodine is released (same as pure iodine)

RADIOACTIVE IODINE (I-131)
- Usually given as a single dose
- Concentrates in thyroid gland and ablates cells
- Infrequent adverse reactions, but may include sore throat and nausea
- Effect of treatment can take 1 to 3 months

PROPRANOLOL
MOA
- Non-selective β-blocker
- β-receptors upregulated in hyperthyroidism
- Antagonizes the cardiovascular and neurological effects resulting from excess adrenergic stimulation

USES
- Provides rapid temporary symptomatic relief (e.g. in thyroid storm)
- Prevents supraventricular arrhythmias
- Not used alone for long-term therapy and is usually discontinued once thyroid levels are stabilized as a result of other treatments

PROPYLTHIOURACIL (PTU)
MOA
- Inhibits addition of iodine to thyroglobulin by the enzyme thyroperoxidase
- Inhibits the peripheral enzyme 5'-deiodinase (tetraiodothyronine 5' deiodinase), which converts T_4 to the active form T_3

USES
- Hyperthyroidism
- Note: used during pregnancy

PK
- Short $t_{1/2}$ (2 hours)

ADRs
- Skin rash (hypersensitivity)
- Bitter taste
- GI discomfort
- Severe liver injury
- Agranulocytosis (rare)
- Aplastic anemia (rare)

METHIMAZOLE
MOA
- Inhibits addition of iodine to thyroglobulin by the enzyme thyroperoxidase

USES
- Hyperthyroidism

PK
- Long $t_{1/2}$ (12 hours)

ADRs
- Skin rash (hypersensitivity)
- Agranulocytosis
- Aplastic anemia
- Bitter taste (less than PTU)
- GI discomfort
- Hepatitis

PERCHLORATE
MOA
- Target = Iodine transport and trapping
- Inhibits trapping
- Inhibit iodine binding and discharge of iodine from thyroid gland

ADRs
- Aplastic anemia + myelosuppression
- Nephrotic syndrome (proteinuria) – iodine disrupts charge barrier
- Gastric irritation
- Nausea, vomiting, fever, rashes

Antidiabetic Drugs

Glucose is required for cellular respiration and survival. Glucose enters the blood after absorption from the gastrointestinal tract or release from the liver (gluconeogenesis and glycogenolysis). Glucose uptake by tissues is regulated by insulin which activates glucose transporters (GLUT = glucose transporter in muscle and fat). Red blood cells, neurons, and the renal medulla absolutely require glucose as a substrate for oxidation (i.e. they cannot burn fat). Regulation of blood glucose levels is important for ensuring systemic glucose delivery but also to prevent the development of many pathologies.

Diabetes is a disease in which glucose homeostasis is impaired resulting in hyperglycemia (fasting glucose $\geq$126mg/dl or 6.1 mmol/L). Prolonged hyperglycemia results in a variety of pathologies, most of which result from non-enzymatic glycation where sugar molecules become covalently linked to proteins. Hemoglobin A1c (HbA1c) levels indicate the degree of non-enzymatic glycosylation and are a good marker over time of how well the patient's blood glucose is being controlled.
  HbA1c primary goal <7%
  HbA1c secondary goal <6%

Main causes of death in Diabetes Mellitus: Cardiovascular disease and kidney failure

Type 1 Diabetes Mellitus (Insulin Dependent Diabetes Mellitus, IDDM)

ASSOCIATIONS
- Usually young (<20 years of age)
- Family history not common
- Sudden onset → polydipsia, polyuria, polyphagia, rapid weight loss
- Severe hyperglycemia
- Ketone bodies in blood

CAUSE
- Autoimmune, or viral associated destruction of pancreatic beta cells
- Decreased plasma insulin (especially after meals)
- Tissues are responsive to insulin

MANAGEMENT
- Exogenous insulin

Review of Insulin Physiology

INSULIN
- Release is stimulated by elevated blood sugar and vagus nerve
- Produced by pancreatic **beta** cells
- Causes muscle and fat to take up glucose from the blood
- Inhibits glycogen breakdown and gluconeogenesis in the liver

GLUCAGON
- Produced by pancreatic **alpha** cells
- Decreases after a meal
- Release is inhibited by elevated blood glucose
- Stimulates liver gluconeogenesis

MECHANISM OF INSULIN RELEASE (like a neural synapse)
1. Glucose enters beta cells → ATP levels rise from elevated glycolysis
2. ATP causes K$^+$ channels to **close**
3. Blocked K$^+$ efflux causes the cell to depolarize
4. Depolarization opens Ca^{2+} channels
5. Ca^{2+} influx causes insulin release from secretory granules

Type 2 Diabetes Mellitus (Non-Insulin Dependent Diabetes Mellitus, NIDDM)

ASSOCIATIONS
- Obesity, hypertension and hyperlipidemia
- Usually older (>30 years of age)
- Very common family history
- Moderate hyperglycemia
- Ketoacidosis (rare)

CAUSE
- Low insulin release combined with insulin resistance of peripheral tissues
- Plasma insulin levels vary

MANAGEMENT
- Weight loss and exercise
- Oral antidiabetics
- Exogenous insulin

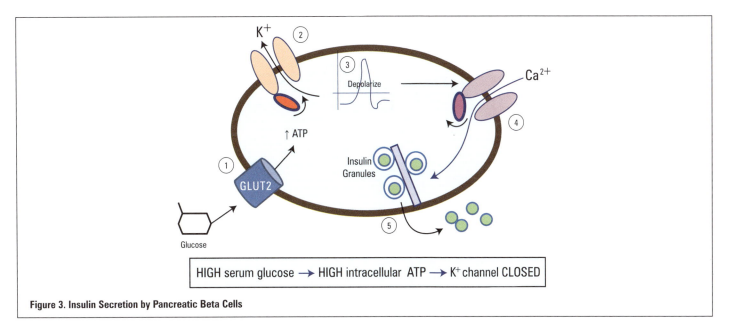

Figure 3. Insulin Secretion by Pancreatic Beta Cells

Antidiabetic Drugs – Type 1

Treatment of Type I Diabetes with Insulin

MOA
1. Insulin binds to the α subunits of the insulin receptor (IR)
2. Intracellular β subunit autophosphorylates tyrosine residues and insulin receptor substrates (IRS-1 and IRS-2)
3. IRS-1 activates several protein kinases leading to translocation of glucose transporters from an intracellular site to the cell membrane

USES
- Type I and 2 DM to try and mimic normal insulin and glucose levels
- Life threatening hyperkalemia
- Stress induced (cortisol) hyperglycemia

ADRs
- **Hypoglycemia** (hunger, sweating, weakness, drowsy, warmth, dizzy, blurred vision, seizures, coma)
  - Symptoms relieved by oral glucose ingestion
  - For severe hypoglycemia, IV glucose and/or glucagon should be administered
  - Hypoglycemia may be asymptomatic in patients who are often hypoglycemic
- **Allergic reactions (rare)**
  - Insulin allergy and resistance
  - May occur with human insulin due to aggregation or denaturation of insulin or components such as protamine added to the formulation
  - Most frequent allergic reactions are IgE-mediated local cutaneous reactions
  - Treated by desensitization with antihistamines for subcutaneous and glucocorticoids for severe systemic reactions
- Lipoatrophy and lipohypertrophy
  - On rare occasions, atrophy of subcutaneous fatty tissue (lipoatrophy) may occur at the site of injection
  - Enlarged subcutaneous fat depots (lipohypertrophy) at the site of repeated injections due to lipogenic action of high local concentrations of insulin
  - Prevented by rotating the injection sites

Insulin Formulations

ASPART
- Ultra short-acting insulin
- Can be given IV and used in insulin pumps

LISPRO
- Ultra-short acting with rapid onset and short duration of action
- Can be given IV and used in insulin pumps

REGULAR
- Short-acting with rapid onset of action
- Can be given IV

NPH
- Intermediate-acting
- Cannot be used IV

GLARGINE
- Peakless, very long-acting with slow onset

DETEMIR
- Peakless, very long-acting with slow onset

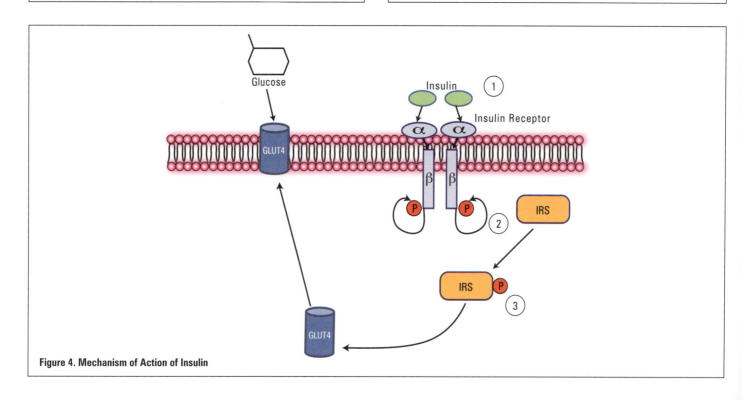

Figure 4. Mechanism of Action of Insulin

Antidiabetic Drugs – Type 2

Oral Drugs for Treatment of Type 2 Diabetes

CAUSES OF TYPE 2 DM (NIDDM)
a. Pancreas does not secreate sufficient insulin in response to glucose
b. Liver secretes excess glucose
c. Receptor and post-receptor insensitivity – muscle does not take up sufficient glucose in response to insulin
d. Most commonly associated with obesity

TREATMENT STRATEGIES
a. Reduce hyperglycemia by strict diet control and exercise program
b. Stimulate the release of insulin from pancreatic beta-cells
c. Increase peripheral insulin sensitivity
d. Decrease hepatic glucose production
e. Inhibit α-glucoside hydrolase and α-amylase in the gut lumen, resulting in delayed absorption and metabolism of carbohydrates
f. Administer insulin as in type 1 diabetes

COMMON SIDE EFFECTS OF ORAL ANTIDIABETIC DRUGS
- Hypoglycemia – especially **GLYBURIDE** and **REPAGLINIDE**
- Weight gain – especially **PIOGLITAZONE**
- These drugs can be used in combination and with insulin, but dose must be titrated to avoid hypoglycemia

Insulin Secretagogues

2nd Generation Sulfonylureas

GLYBURIDE
MOA
- Stimulates insulin release from pancreas
- Blocks K^+ ATP channel beta-cells → depolarization → Ca^{2+} channels open → insulin release by exocytosis
- Used for type 2 DM only - requires residual islet function

PK
- Moderate $t_{1/2}$ (10 hours)
- Duration of action is 18-24 hours

ADRs
- **Hypoglycemia**
- Weight gain
- Sulfa allergy
- Bad taste in mouth
- GI discomfort
- Blood dyscrasias
- Liver toxicity (cholestatic jaundice)
- Disulfiram reaction

Meglitinides

REPAGLINIDE
MOA
- Binds unique receptor → K^+ channels close → insulin released

PK
- Short $t_{1/2}$ (1-4 hours)
- Duration of action is 4-5 hours

ADRs
- No disulfiram-like reaction
- Hypoglycemia (less than glyburide since shorter duration of action)
- Weight gain

Drugs that Inhibit Sugar Absorption

ACARBOSE
MOA
- Inhibits α-glucoside hydrolase and α-amylase in the gut lumen
  - → Delay postprandial glucose absorption

PK
- Short $t_{1/2}$ (2 hours)
- Duration of action is 4-5 hours

ADRs
- Liver toxicity → increased LFT values
- GI discomfort – osmotic diarrhea

Insulin Sensitizers

Thiazolidinediones

PIOGLITAZONE, ROSIGLITAZONE
MOA
1. Activate the PPARγ nuclear receptor
2. Increases the number of GLUT4 in adipose and muscle cells (via increased transcription) → increased glucose uptake
3. Increases fat synthesis and storage
4. Decreases hepatic glucose production

PK
- Moderate $t_{1/2}$ (3-7 hours)
- Duration of action is 10-24 hours

ADRs
- Causes the most weight gain of all diabetic therapeutics
- Increased blood cholesterol
- Cardiovascular effects → fluid accumulation/retention
  - Especially when used in combination with insulin increases risk of heart failure
  - **ROSIGLITAZONE** is associated with increased risk of myocardial infarction
- Mild to moderate edema
- Anemia
- Hepatotoxic

Biguanides

METFORMIN
MOA
- Decreases hepatic glucose production by inhibiting gluconeogenesis
- Increases glucose uptake from blood
  - Makes insulin receptor more sensitive in adipose, liver and muscle cells

PK
- Short $t_{1/2}$ (1.7-3 hours)
- Duration of action is 10-12 hours

ADRs
- Lactic acidosis (especially during renal insufficiency) → increased anion gap
- GI discomfort
- Alteration of taste
- Megaloblastic anemia

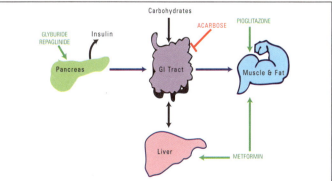

Figure 5. Therapeutics Used to Treat Type 2 Diabetes Mellitus

Corticosteroids

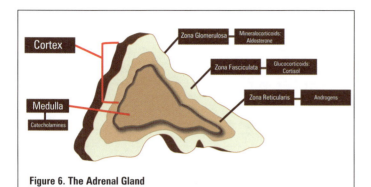

Figure 6. The Adrenal Gland

Steroids Made in the Adrenal Cortex

Corticosteroids (21C)
1) Mineralocorticoids (aldosterone)
2) Glucocorticoids (cortisol)

Androgens (19C)
1) Dehydroepiandrosterone (DHEA)
2) Androstenedione
3) Testosterone

Zona glomerulosa
1) Produces aldosterone
2) Regulated by renin-angiotensin system and potassium
3) Express steroid 11β-monooxygenase (aldosterone synthase, CYP11B2 isozyme)

Zona fasciculata/reticularis
1) Produces glucocorticoids (cortisol) and androgens
2) Regulated by ACTH
3) Express steroid 17α-monooxygenase and steroid 11β-monooxygenase (CYP11B1 isozyme)

- Insignificant source of androgens in males
- Significant source of testosterone and estradiol in post-menopausal women
- EXCESS androgen synthesis from adrenal cortex → VIRILIZATION in men and women

The Hypothalamic-Pituitary-Adrenal Axis

ADENOCORTICOTROPIC HORMONE (ACTH)
- Regulates corticosteroid biosynthesis and release

MOA
- Binds to a cell membrane receptor that activates adenylyl cyclase → increases cAMP, resulting in cAMP-dependent increase in transcription of genes encoding steroidogenic enzymes

USES
- Clinical diagnostic test for adrenal insufficiency
- Assess adrenal response to stimulation from the pituitary

PK
- Very short $t_{1/2}$ (15 minutes)

PHYSIOLOGIC EFFECTS
- Mainly in zona reticularis and fasciculata
- Increases cholesterol uptake into cells and mitochondria, and stimulates conversion of cholesterol to pregnenolone (RLS!) → increased production of cortisol
- Some effect to stimulate production and release of aldosterone in the zona glomerulosa of the adrenal cortex
- Stimulates growth of the adrenal cortex
- Lack of ACTH → degeneration of the zona fasciculata/reticularis

Corticosteroid Biosynthesis

Rate Limiting Step (RLS): Cholesterol is converted by cholesterol monooxygenase (desmolase, CYP11A1) to **pregnenolone** (a ketone)

Ⓐ 17-α-monooxygenase (CYP17)
- Converts pregnenolone to 17-α-hydroxypregnenolone

The next three conversions to cortisol are mediated by:
3-β-hydroxysteroid-dehydrogenase (HSD3B1) (17-hydroxypregnenolone → 17-α-hydroxyprogesterone)
Ⓑ 21-monooxygenase (CYP21B2)
Ⓒ 11-β-monooxygenase (CYP11B1)

The same mechanism is used to make aldosterone with an additional step by **aldosterone synthase**

Adrenal corticosteroids are not stored in the adrenal gland, therefore their rate of synthesis equals their rate of secretion.
The blood serves as the reservoir for corticosteroids.

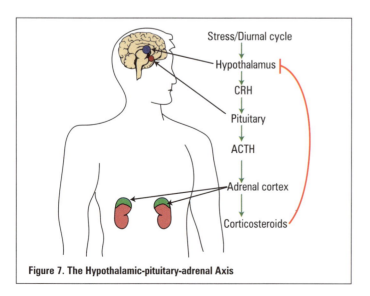

Figure 7. The Hypothalamic-pituitary-adrenal Axis

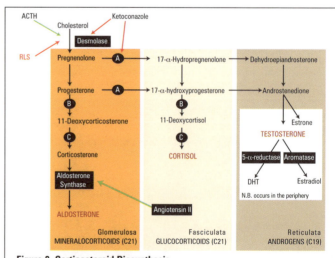

Figure 8. Corticosteroid Biosynthesis

Corticosteroids

MOA
- Corticosteroids enter the cell, bind to cytosolic corticosteroid receptors that transport the steroids into the nucleus
- The steroid-receptor complex alters gene expression by binding to glucocorticoid response elements (GRE)
- Tissue-specific responses to steroids are regulated by the presence of different protein regulators that control the interaction between the hormone-receptor complex and particular response element
- In mineralocorticoid target tissues, 11β-hydroxysteroid dehydrogenase (11β-HSD) inactivates glucocorticoids, making these tissues predominantly responsive to mineralcorticoids

PHYSIOLOGIC EFFECTS
Permissive Effects
- The action of catecholamines on vascular and bronchial smooth muscle requires the presence of cortisol

Three Major Physiologic Effects
1. Essential for homeostasis and coping with stress
2. Influence carbohydrate, protein, and lipid metabolism (glucocorticoids)
3. Maintain homeostasis of several systems
   - Mineralocorticoids – electrolyte and water balance
   - Aldosterone – renal Na^+ and water reabsorption in the DCT and collecting ducts

Nonspecific Effects
- Glucocorticoids have some mineralocorticoid activity and mineralcorticoids have some glucocorticoid activity

USES
- Diagnosis and treatment of primary or secondary adrenal hyper/hypofunctions
- Prevention of infant respiratory distress syndrome
  - Maternal treatment between 24-34 weeks for preterm delivery
- Anti-inflammatory and immune suppression
- Rheumatoid arthritis, autoimmune disease, allergic diseases, bronchial asthma, many topical dermatological uses, high altitude pulmonary or cerebral edema
- Corticosteroids are not curative – only suppress symptoms, does not treat underlying cause

ADRs
- Fluid electrolyte disturbances (esp. **ALDOSTERONE**)
- Hyperglycemia and glycosuria (esp. **CORTISOL**)
- Increase susceptibility to infection
- Peptic ulcers – *H. pylori*
- Thrush, if taken orally
- Osteoporosis
- Cushing's syndrome
- Proximal myopathy and muscle wasting
- Hypomania or acute psychosis, depression
- Subcapsular cataracts
- Glucocorticoids, in excess, cause hypertension independent of mineralocorticoids
- Glucocorticoid withdrawal may result in adrenal insufficiency causing:
  - Anorexia, nausea and vomiting, weight loss, fever, malaise, myalgia

Diseases of Hypo- or Hyper- Cortisolemia

Adrenal Insufficiency (cortisol and aldosterone insufficiency)
(salt wasting, fatigue, orthostatic hypotension, hyperpigmentation)
- Due to primary adrenal cortex dysfunction (ACTH is high)
  - Idiopathic
  - Autoimmune (**Addison's Disease**)
  - Adenoma
- Secondary to pituitary dysfunction (ACTH is inappropriately low)

Cushing's Syndrome (hypercortisolemia)
(moon fascies, dorsal fat pad, abdominal striae, abdominal adiposity)
- **Exogenous**
  - Usually caused by exogenous glucocorticoid administration
- **Endogenous**
  - Primary: hypersecretion of cortisol in adrenal cortex (ACTH low)
  - Secondary: hypersecretion due to high ACTH

Key Causes of Cushing's Syndrome: Pituitary adenoma (Cushing's disease), ectopic ACTH, adrenal adenoma, ectopic glucocorticoids

Glucocorticoids

CORTISOL

Regulators of Cortisol Release
- Physiologic secretion is regulated by ACTH and varies during the day
- Has a small but significant salt-retaining (mineralocorticoid) effect
  - This causes the hypertension associated with cortisol-secreting adrenal tumor or pituitary ACTH secreting tumor (Cushing's syndrome)

Glucocorticoid-specific Actions (receptors are ubiquitous)
- Glucose, fat, protein
  - Increase serum glucose and liver glycogen
    - Increase enzymes for converting amino acids → glucose
    - Stimulate glycogen synthase in the liver
    - Stimulates amino acid mobilization from muscle
- Increased glucose levels increase insulin release
  - Causes insulin resistance in muscle and fat
  - Decrease protein synthesis, but stimulate it in the liver
  - Stimulate lipolysis in fat → higher blood fatty acids
  - BUT, cortisol → higher glucose → insulin which causes more fat synthesis → fattening in the face, neck, and trunk (central obesity)
- Anti-inflammatory
  - Inhibits cytokine, chemokine and lipid mediators of inflammation
  - Increase neutrophils and decrease all other WBCs
  - Decreases responsiveness of leukocytes and macrophages

PK
- Short $t_{1/2}$ (1.5 hours)

Mineralocorticoids

ALDOSTERONE

Regulators of Aldosterone Release
- Renin-angiotensin system
- Regulators of aldosterone release
  - High plasma $[K^+]$ (most potent regulator)
  - Low plasma $[Na^+]$
- ACTH has a permissive effect on aldosterone

Aldosterone-Specific Actions
- Receptors restricted to locations involving water/thirst:
  - DCT and collecting ducts of kidney
  - Colon
  - Sweat glands
  - Hippocampus
- Functions to promote:
  - Na^+ and HCO_3^- retention
  - K^+ secretion

Consequences of No Aldosterone
- High K^+, low Na^+, low Cl^- in plasma
- Reduced ECV and blood volume
- High K^+ → cardiotoxicity

Consequences of High Aldosterone
- Na^+ retention → fluid retention and increased drinking NOT an increase in plasma $[Na^+]$
- K^+ loss → hypokalemia → muscle cramp/weakness

PK
- Short $t_{1/2}$ (15-30 minutes)

Corticosteroids

Synthetic Mineralocorticosteroids

FLUDROCORTISONE
MOA
- Identical to **ALDOSTERONE**
- Mineralocorticoid action is much greater than anti-inflammatory action

USES
- Causes Na+ and fluid retention
- Hypoaldosteronism replacement therapy

Mineralocorticoid Antagonists

SPIRONOLACTONE
Note: See Renal and Urological Drugs chapter

MOA
- Aldosterone receptor antagonist
- Potassium sparing diuretic
- Na+ and water are lost when it is administered
- Requires the presence of aldosterone
- Greatest utility in hyperaldosteronism to minimize K+ loss

Adrenocortical Synthesis Blockers
Synthesis Inhibitors and Glucocorticoid Antagonists

AMINOGLUTETHIMIDE
MOA
- Non-selective agent that inhibits desmolase (CYP11A1) and steroid 11-β monooxygenase (CYP11B1) to block the initial and rate-limiting step in the biosynthesis of all physiological steroids

USES
- Treat Cushing's syndrome
  - Secondary to adrenal carcinoma
  - Ectopic production of ACTH

METYRAPONE
MOA
- Inhibits steroid 11-β-monooxygenase in the adrenal cortex and hence cortisol and corticosterone synthesis

USES
- Diagnostic test and treatment for Cushing's syndrome

KETOCONAZOLE
MOA
- Inhibits 17-β-monooxygenase (CYP17) and desmolase (CYP11A1) (at high doses)

USES
- Cushing's syndrome
- antifungal (see Antimicrobial Drugs chapter)

Synthetic Glucocorticosteroids

MOA
- Identical to that of cortisol

USES
- Addison's disease
- Immune suppression/anti-inflammatory
- Asthma

ADRs
- Iatrogenic Cushing's syndrome (most common cause of Cushing's syndrome)

HYDROCORTISONE
USES
- Preferred drug for replacement therapy
- Commonly used as a topical anti-inflammatory, but NOT useful as a systemic anti-inflammatory agent because its anti-inflammatory and salt-retaining actions are equal

PK
- Short $t_{1/2}$ (1-2 hours)

PREDNISONE
USES
- Good choice for CHRONIC anti-inflammatory therapy (asthma) because of increased anti-inflammatory potency and decreased mineralocorticoid potency

PK
- Very long $t_{1/2}$ (12-36 hours)

BETAMETHASONE and DEXAMETHASONE
USES
- Anti-inflammatory effect only
- Good choice for ACUTE anti-inflammatory therapy
- NOT first choice for chronic treatment due to growth suppression and bone demineralization

PK
- Very long $t_{1/2}$ (36-54 hours)

NOTE
- Dexamethasone test distinguishes between ectopic ACTH and ACTH released from the pituitary. Ectopic (i.e. small cell lung cancer) ACTH will not decrease upon a dexamethasone challenge because it originates from outside the hypothalamic-pituitary-adrenal axis

Compound	Anti-inflammatory Potency	Na+-Retaining Potency	Duration of Action*
Cortisone	0.8	0.8	Short
Fludrocortisone	10	125	Intermediate
Prednisone	4	0.8	Intermediate
Betamethasone	25	0	Long
Dexamethasone	25	0	Long

*Short – 8-12 h biological $t_{1/2}$
Intermediate – 12-36 h biological $t_{1/2}$
Long – 36-72 h biological $t_{1/2}$

Gastrointestinal Drugs

Chapter Authors: Andrew W. Browne, Jeeyeon M. Cha and Janine R. Hutson

Faculty Reviewers: Samir C. Grover and Geert W. 't Jong

IN THIS CHAPTER

Introduction	116
Anti-Bloating Drugs	116
Inflammatory Bowel Disease	117
Anti-Diarrheals	118
Laxatives	119
Anti-Emetics	120
Peptic Ulcer Disease and GERD	122

DRUGS IN THIS CHAPTER

Generic Name	US Trade Name	Canadian Trade Name
5-aminosalicylic acid	ASACOL, CANASA, PENTASA, ROWASA, LIALDA, APRISO	ASACOL, MESASAL, MEZAVANT, PENTASA, SALOFALK
aluminum hydroxide, magnesium hydroxide	ALAMAG, MAALOX, KUDROX	MAALOX, UNIVOL, DIOVO
aprepitant	EMEND	
bisacodyl	DULCOLAX, CORRECTOL, DOXIDAN, BISCOLAX, ALOPHEN	BI-PEGLYTE, CARTERS LITTLE PILLS, DULCOLAX
bismuth subsalicylate	PEPTO-BISMOL	
calcium carbonate	ROLAIDS, TUMS, CALTRATE	
castor oil	PURGE	
cimetidine	TAGAMET	
diphenoxylate	LOMOCOT, LOMOTIL, LONOX	LOMOTIL
docusate	COLACE, DIOCTO, DIOSUCCIN	SOFLAX, COLACE, SELAX
domperidone		
dronabinol	MARINOL	
famotidine	PEPCID	
infliximab	REMICADE	
ipecac syrup		
loperamide	DIAMODE, IMODIUM, IMOGEN, IMOTIL, IMPERIM	IMODIUM
magnesium salts		
methylcellulose		
metoclopramide	REGLAN, METOZOLV	REGLAN
misoprostol	CYTOTEC	ARTHROTEC
nizatidine	AXID	
octreotide	SANDOSTATIN	
olsalazine	DIPENTUM	
omeprazole	PRILOSEC	LOSEC
ondansetron	ZOFRAN, ZUPLENZ	ZOFRAN
polyethylene glycol	GAVILAX, GLYCOLAX, MIRALAX	COLYTE, KLEAN-PREP, LAX-A-DAY, PEGALAX, PEGLYTE
prochlorperazine	COMPAZINE, COMPRO	
psyllium	METAMUCIL	
ranitidine	ZANTAC, TALADINE	ZANTAC
simethicone	MYLICON, GAS X, MYLANTA GAS, GENASYME, MYTAB GAS, PHAZYME	DIVOL PLUS, GAS X, MYLANTA GAS, OVOL, PHAZYME
sucralfate	CARAFATE	SULCRATE
sulfasalazine	AZULFIDINE, SULFAZINE	SALAZOPYRIN

Introduction

Non-infectious disturbances in the gastrointestinal (GI) tract that are treated pharmacologically fall into 3 categories:

1. Disturbances in Motility
   - Common GI conditions such as nausea, vomiting, diarrhea, delayed gastric emptying and constipation
   - Laxatives, anti-diarrheals and anti-flatulents are among the most common drugs purchased over the counter (OTC)
   - It is important to investigate the cause of these common GI symptoms as they could be related to primary GI conditions or secondary symptoms to primary conditions in other systems
     - GI therapeutics may mask or worsen the underlying condition
     - For example, in sufficient doses, all opioids have constipation as an adverse drug reaction. Constipation in patients using opioids may be a reason to check for overdosing or abuse

2. Inflammatory Bowel Disease (IBD)
   - IBD, which is comprised of Crohn's disease and ulcerative colitis, can be a cause of rectal bleeding, weight loss, diarrhea, and many other GI symptoms. Treatment of these conditions typically involves anti-inflammatory medications and immunosuppressants

3. Acid-peptic disorders
   - The pathophysiology of many upper GI disorders are caused by gastric acid and pepsin. These can become pathogenic when either:
     i. *H. pylori* infection causes ↑ secretion
     ii. Other conditions ↓ mucosal protection from gastric acid or pepsin (e.g. chronic NSAID use)
   - A common cause of upper GI ulcers is gastroesophageal reflux disease (GERD), which can be managed by non-pharmacologic strategies. When ulcers are severe, however, pharmacologic interventions may be employed, such as anti-bacterials, acid neutralizing agents, and cytoprotective agents

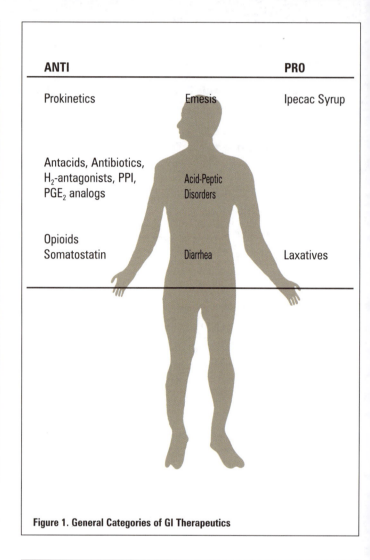

Figure 1. General Categories of GI Therapeutics

Anti-Bloating Drugs

SIMETHICONE

MOA
- ↓ surface tension of gas bubbles and cause smaller bubbles to aggregate into larger bubbles
- ↑ rate of gas exiting the body

USES
- Excessive upper gastrointestinal gas
- Preparation for imaging
- Flatulence

PK
- Not absorbed

ADRs
- Diarrhea
- Nausea

Inflammatory Bowel Disease

Ulcerative Colitis

- Autoimmune etiology
- Affects the colon only, continuously from the rectum
- Complications: toxic megacolon, colorectal cancer
- Treatment: 5-ASA, immunosuppressants, colectomy

Crohn's Disease

- Multifactorial etiology
- Can affect the entire GI tract with skip lesions and transmural inflammation
- Complications: malabsorption, fistulas
- Treatment: Steroids, immunosuppressants

Anti-Inflammatory Agents

5-AMINOSALICYLIC ACID (5-ASA)
SULFASALAZINE
OLSALAZINE

MOA
- Inhibits prostaglandin and leukotriene production in gut

USES
- Crohn's disease
- Ulcerative colitis
- Indeterminate colitis
- Rheumatoid arthritis (SULFASALAZINE)

PK 5-ASA
- Short $t_{1/2}$ (< 1 hour)

PK SULFASALAZINE
- Moderate $t_{1/2}$ (7 hours)

PK OLSALAZINE
- Short $t_{1/2}$ (1 hour)

ADRs
- Malaise
- Nausea, abdominal discomfort
- Sulfonamide sensitivity (hypersensitivity reaction)
- Folic acid deficiency (5-ASA)
- Hepatotoxicity (5-ASA)
- Yellow-orange discolored urine (SULFASALAZINE)

Immunosuppression

Corticosteroids
- e.g. HYDROCORTISONE, PREDNISONE (see Immune Response Modifiers chapter)

Cytotoxic Agents
- e.g. AZATHIOPRINE, MERCAPTOPURINE (see Cancer Chemotherapeutics chapter)

Monoclonal Antibody

INFLIXIMAB

MOA
- Neutralizes TNFα

USES
- Crohn's disease
- Ulcerative colitis
- Rheumatoid arthritis
- Psoriasis
- Ankylosing spondylitis

PK
- Very long $t_{1/2}$ (9-10 days)

ADRs
- Nausea, abdominal pain
- Headache
- Fatigue
- Respiratory tract infections
- Reactivation of tuberculosis or chronic hepatitis B

Anti-Diarrheals

Opioids

LOPERAMIDE

MOA
- Opioid agonist
- Slows intestinal motility and increases sphincter tone

USES
- Acute and chronic diarrhea
- Traveler's diarrhea

PK
- Moderate $t_{1/2}$ (10 hours)

ADRs
- Dizziness
- Abdominal pain
- Fatigue
- Constipation

CONTRAINDICATIONS
- Pseudomembranous colitis

DIPHENOXYLATE

MOA
- Opioid agonist
- ↓ peristalsis
- Counteracts excessive secretion

USES
- Self-limited diarrhea or mild chronic diarrhea

PK
- Short $t_{1/2}$ (2-4 hours)

ADRs
- Abdominal discomfort
- Sedation
- Euphoria

Somatostatin Analogs

OCTREOTIDE

MOA
- Analogue of **SOMATOSTATIN** → inhibits secretion of:
  - Acid
  - Pepsinogen
  - Bicarbonate
- Inhibition of gastrin and other peptide hormones
- ↓ smooth muscle contractility

USES
- Treatment of refractory diarrhea
- Idiopathic diarrhea of AIDS or the elderly
- Diarrhea associated with vasoactive intestinal peptide-secreting tumor

PK
- Short $t_{1/2}$ (2 hours)

ADRs
- Gallstone formation
- Injection site irritation
- Constipation
- Impaired glucose homeostasis

Laxatives

Saline/Osmotics

MAGNESIUM SALTS

MOA
- Non-absorbable hypertonic ions retain fluid in the gut lumen due to osmotic action
- Increase rate of transit in the small intestine

ADRs
- Electrolyte imbalance
- Dehydration

NOTES
- Watery stool produced rapidly (1-3 hours after administration)

POLYETHYLENE GLYCOL

MOA
- Osmotic agent that causes water retention in the stool
- Results in softer stool and more frequent bowel movements

USES
- Constipation
- Whole bowel irrigation prior to surgery or colonoscopy
- Whole bowel irrigation after toxic ingestion

ADRs
- Electrolyte imbalance
- Stomach cramps

Stimulants

BISACODYL

MOA
- ↑ parasympathetic reflexes leading to ↑ peristaltic contractions of the colon
- ↑ intestinal fluid by altering water and electrolyte secretion

ADRs
- Abdominal cramping
- Proctitis (with rectal suppository)

CONTRAINDICATIONS
- Appendicitis
- Gastroenteritis

NOTES
- Onset of action is 6-8 hours after oral administration
- More rapid onset when given in a rectal suppository (1 hour)

CASTOR OIL

MOA
- Stimulant laxative
- Hydrolyzed by pancreatic lipases to glycerol and ricinoleic acid

ADRs
- Electrolyte imbalance
- Abdominal pain
- Nausea
- Vomiting

CONTRAINDICATIONS
- Abdominal pain
- Symptoms of appendicitis
- Nausea, vomiting

NOTES
- May also be used as a purgative

Dietary Fiber/Bulk Forming Agents

PSYLLIUM, METHYLCELLULOSE

MOA
- ↑ stool mass, which stimulates peristalsis
- ↑ water content of stool

ADRs
- Abdominal distention

NOTES
- Soft stool produced in 1-3 days (slower-acting laxative)
- Concurrent administration of fluids is recommended

Emolient/Lubricant (Stool Softener)

DOCUSATE CALCIUM, DOCUSATE SODIUM

MOA
- Draws water into the stool

USES
- Prevents straining at the toilet (Valsalva maneuver)

ADRs
- Abnormal/bitter taste in mouth
- Abdominal cramps
- Diarrhea
- Intestinal obstruction
- Muscle cramps
- Throat irritation

DRUG INTERACTIONS
- Mineral oil
- May alter absorption of other drugs – should not take within 2 hours of other medications

NOTES
- Soft stool produced in 1-3 days (slower-acting laxative)
- Minimally effective, especially in chronic constipation
- Additional example: glycerin suppository

Use of Laxatives

Generally, laxatives are used for the following:
- Uncomplicated constipation
- Preparation for a GI examination
- Prevention of straining in cardiac patients
- Hemorrhoids
- Post-operative constipation

Laxatives should not be used when there is possible bowel obstruction, habitual use of laxatives, or irritable bowel. Stimulant laxatives are popular and are often abused.

Anti-Emetics

Emesis

Emesis is controlled by the emetic centers in the brain stem. Afferents to the emetic center arrive from the Central (CNS) and Peripheral (PNS) Nervous Systems. When the emetic center is stimulated, efferent pathways to end effector organs result in salivation, decreased respiration and emesis.

IPECAC SYRUP
- Pro-emetic
- Rarely used to induce emesis after recent toxic ingestion

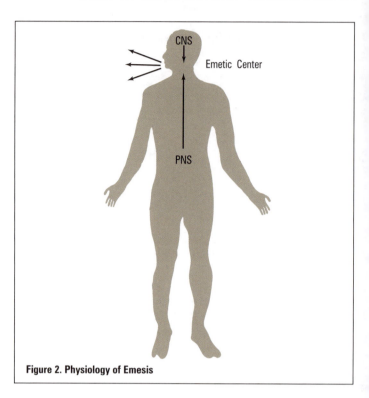

Figure 2. Physiology of Emesis

Prokinetic Agents

METOCLOPRAMIDE
MOA
- Stimulates 5-HT$_4$ receptors
- Acts both centrally and peripherally
  - Peripheral
    - Sensitizes tissues to ACh
  - Central
    - Stimulates upper GI tract motility without affecting secretions and independent of intact vagal innervation
    - Raises lower esophageal pressure and enhances gastric emptying
    - D$_2$-receptor antagonist → blocks medullary chemoreceptor trigger zone

USES
- Anti-emetic
- Chemotherapy induced nausea/vomiting
- GERD
- Diabetic and post-surgery gastroparesis

PK
- Moderate t$_{1/2}$ (5 hours)

ADRs
- Fatigue/drowsiness
- Dizziness
- Fluid retention
- Parkinsonian effects from dopamine blockade
- Cardiac arrhythmia
- Gynecomastia (with chronic use due to increased prolactin)

DOMPERIDONE
MOA
- Peripheral D$_1$- and D$_2$-receptor antagonist
- Increases gastric emptying, esophageal peristalsis and lower esophageal sphincter tone

USES
- Anti-emetic
- Anti-nauseant

PK
- Moderate t$_{1/2}$ (8 hours)

ADRs
- Galactorrhea
- Menstrual irregularities
- Headache
- Abdominal cramps

NOTES
- Fewer side effects compared to **METOCLOPRAMIDE** since does not easily cross the BBB
- In infants, however, overdosing may lead to neurological side effects

Anti-Emetics

Centrally Acting Anti-Emetics

PROCHLORPERAZINE
MOA
- In the phenothiazine class and is a typical antipsychotic
- Central
  - Dopamine antagonist in the medullary chemoreceptor trigger zone
- Peripheral
  - Blocks the vagus nerve in the GI tract

USES
- Anti-emetic
- Anxiety
- Schizophrenia

PK
- Moderate $t_{1/2}$ (8 hours)

ADRs
- Hypotension
- Extrapyramidal symptoms
- Blurred vision
- Constipation

ONDANSETRON
MOA
- 5-HT_3-receptor antagonist to block vagal stimulation by serotonin

USES
- Post-operative emesis
- Chemotherapy induced nausea/vomiting

PK
- Moderate $t_{1/2}$ (5 hours)

ADRs
- Fatigue
- Headache
- Constipation or diarrhea
- Cardiac dysrhythmia

APREPITANT
MOA
- Neurokinin 1 (NK1) antagonist

USES
- Chemotherapy induced nausea/vomiting
- Post-operative nausea/vomiting

PK
- Moderate $t_{1/2}$ (10 hours)

ADRs
- Fatigue
- Diarrhea
- Sinus tachycardia
- Dizziness

DRONABINOL
MOA
- Unknown mechanism
  - Likely due to cannabinoid receptor activity

USES
- Chemotherapy induced nausea/vomiting

PK
- Long $t_{1/2}$ (20 hours)

ADRs
- Flushing
- Dry mouth
- Euphoria
- Somnolence
- Increased appetite

Other Anti-Emetics

1st Generation Antihistamines
DIMENHYDRINATE
CHLORPHENYRAMINE
PROMETHAZINE
DOXYLAMINE (in combination with **PYRIDOXINE** for nausea and vomiting in pregnancy)

Anticholinergics
ATROPINE
SCOPOLAMINE

Herbal
Ginger

Peptic Ulcer Disease and GERD

Common causes for gastric ulcers include *H. pylori* infection and chronic GERD

NON-PHARMACOLOGICAL TREATMENT OF GERD
- Diet
  - Small meals, low fat foods
  - Avoid spicy foods, carbonated beverages, chocolate and excess alcohol
- Smoking cessation
- Sleep with head slightly elevated
  - Avoid sleeping immediately after eating (stay upright during digestion)

PHARMACOLOGICAL TREATMENT OF GERD AND GASTRIC ULCERS
- Antibacterial – eliminate *H. pylori* in order to cure chronic peptic ulcer disease
- Neutralization/inhibition of gastric acid – antacids, H_2 antagonists and proton pump inhibitors
- Increased mucus secretion and cytoprotection

Helicobacter pylori

- *H. pylori* is implicated in the vast majority of GERD
- Chronic *H. pylori* infection can lead to:
  - Peptic ulcer disease
  - Chronic superficial gastritis
  - Lymphoproliferative disease
  - Chronic atrophic gastritis → gastric adenocarcinoma

H. Pylori Triple Therapy
- Proton pump inhibitor + 2 antibiotics

COMMON COMBINATIONS

OMEPRAZOLE + CLARITHROMYCIN + AMOXICILLIN

OMEPRAZOLE + METRONIDAZOLE + TETRACYCLINE

BISMUTH SUCRALFATE may be added

Cytoprotective Agents

SUCRALFATE
MOA
- Basic salt of sucrose sulfate and aluminum hydroxide
- Combines with protein exudates at the base of the ulcer and forms a thick paste-like barrier for more than 5 hours
- Does not combine with normal tissue
- No acid-neutralizing capacity but reduces pepsin activity

USES
- GI ulcers and erosions

PK
- Not absorbed

ADRs
- Constipation
- Aluminum toxicity in patients with renal failure

BISMUTH SUBSALICYLATE
MOA
- May stimulate fluid absorption and decrease secretions
- Hydolyzed to salicylic acid to inhibit prostaglandin formation → decreases inflammation and hypermotility
- Metabolites produced in the intestine may have direct bactericidal action
- Provides a protective layer by inhibiting pepsin and increasing mucus production

USES
- Treatment of *H. pylori* infection
- Nausea
- Diarrhea
- Indigestion
- Heartburn

PK
- Very minimal absorption

ADRs
- Constipation/diarrhea
- Abnormal stool color (gray/black)
- Tongue discoloration
- Neurotoxicity (rare)

Mucus Secretion

- Mucus and bicarbonate protect cells in the GI tract
- E- series prostaglandin receptors (PGEs) stimulate their production

Prostaglandin Analogs

MISOPROSTOL
MOA
- Prostaglandin analog (of PGE_1)
- A combination of anti-secretory and cytoprotective effects
  - The gastric mucosa synthesizes PGE_2 and PGI_2 which inhibit basal and stimulated acid secretion regardless of the stimulus by inhibiting adenylate cyclase
  - Enhances the protective mucosal barrier by stimulation of secretion of mucus and bicarbonate

USES
- Prevention of NSAID-induced ulcers
- Can be given with RU-486 (mifepristone) to induce abortion
- Cervical ripening to facilitate labor

PK
- Short $t_{1/2}$ (<1 hour)

ADRs
- Diarrhea
- Abdominal pain
- Flatulence
- Menstrual spotting

Peptic Ulcer Disease and GERD

Acid Secretion

Stimuli
- ACh and gastrin → increased Ca^{2+} → increased acid secretion
- H_2-receptor → increased cAMP → increased acid secretion

Methods to decrease acid (H^+) secretion
- Antagonize receptors
  - Muscarinic (isotype 2 is most important)
  - H_2-receptor
  - Gastrin (causes parietal cells to release acid)
  - Proton pump
- Inhibit secretion
  - PGE_2 → decreased cAMP

RECALL THE DIFFERENT HISTAMINE RECEPTORS
1. H_1 → G_q → activates phospholipase C → increase IP_3+DAG → increase in Ca^{2+}
2. H_2 → G_s → activates adenylate cyclase → increase in cAMP
3. H_3 → $G_{i/o}$ → INHIBITS phospholipase C → decrease in Ca^{2+}

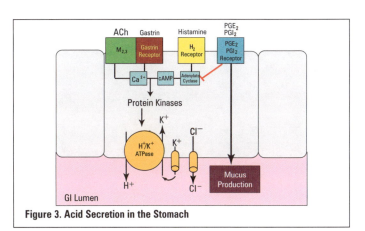

Figure 3. Acid Secretion in the Stomach

H_2-receptor Antagonists

H_2-receptor Mechanism of Action
- H_2-receptors associate with intracellular G proteins
- $G\alpha_s$ activates adenylyl cyclase activity
- Intracellular cAMP increases

H_2-receptor Locations
- Stomach parietal cells – gastric acid production (ulcers)
- Small intestine – increased bicarbonate, pancreatic enzymes
- Heart muscle cells – positive inotropic and chronotropic effect
- Mast cells – decreased mediator release
- Brain – neurons
- Vascular smooth muscle – relaxation, dilation

FAMOTIDINE, CIMETIDINE, RANITIDINE, NIZATIDINE
MOA
- Reversible-competitive antagonists of H_2-receptors of gastric mucosal parietal cells → reduce gastric acid and pepsin production

USES
- Heart burn and ulcers
  - Reduces gastric acid secretions
  - Aids healing of erosive esophagitis
- Treatment of **Zollinger-Ellison Syndrome**, systemic mastocytosis, multiple endocrine adenoma syndrome

PK
FAMOTIDINE
- Short $t_{1/2}$ (3-4 hours)

CIMETIDINE
- Short $t_{1/2}$ (2 hours)

RANITIDINE, NIZATIDINE
- Short $t_{1/2}$ (1-2 hours)

ADRs
- For **CIMETIDINE** only
  - Impotence
  - CYP450 inhibition

Antacids

CALCIUM CARBONATE
MOA
- Neutralization of gastric acid
- Decrease pepsin activity

USES
- Ulcer relief (not cure)
- Alternative or adjunct to H_2-receptor antagonist
- Calcium supplement (prophylaxis against osteoporosis)

PK
- Rapid onset, acts locally

ADRs
- Hypercalcemia (excessive use)
- Hypokalemia
- Systemic alkalosis and phosphate imbalance
- Gastric rebound acid secretion due to local effect of Ca^{2+}
- Chalky taste
- Belching

ALUMINUM HYDROXIDE
- ADRs: constipation, muscle weakness, seizures

MAGNESIUM HYDROXIDE
- ADRs: diarrhea, cardiac arrhythmias

Proton Pump Inhibitors (PPIs)
(names end with "-prazole")

OMEPRAZOLE
MOA
- Selective inhibitor of the H^+/K^+ ATPase of parietal cells
- Suppresses acid secretion under basal conditions and in response to feeding, gastrin, histamine, and vagal stimulation
- Capable of completely blocking acid secretion

USES
- GERD
- Duodenal and gastric ulcer
- *H. pylori* infection
- Zollinger-Ellison syndrome

PK
- Short $t_{1/2}$ (1 hour; the duration of the effect is longer due to irreversible binding to drug target)

ADRs
- Headache, abdominal pain, nausea
- Risk of community acquired pneumonia
  - Chronic use may lead to insufficient elimination of ingested pathogens which then may be aspirated → community-acquired pneumonia

NOTES
- Most efficacious drug for inhibiting acid secretion
- Other PPIs include **PANTOPRAZOLE, LANSOPRAZOLE, RABEPRAZOLE, ESOMEPRAZOLE, DEXLANSOPRAZOLE**

Hematological Drugs

Chapter Authors: Brian G. Ballios and Andrew W. Browne

Faculty Reviewer: Susan Belo

IN THIS CHAPTER

Hemostasis and Erythropoiesis	126
Thrombolytics	127
Anticoagulants	128
Antiplatelet Drugs	130

DRUGS IN THIS CHAPTER

Generic Name	US Trade Name	Canadian Trade Name
abciximab	REOPRO	
alteplase	ACTIVASE, CATHFLO ACTIVASE	
aminocaproic acid	AMICAR	
anistreplase	EMINASE	
aspirin	ECOTRIN, BAYER, ASCRIPTIN, ASPERGUM, ASPIRTAB, EASPRIN, ECPIRIN, ENTERCOTE	ASPIRIN
bivalirudin	ANGIOMAX	
clopidrogel	PLAVIX	
darbepoetin alfa	ARANESP	
enoxaparin	LOVENOX	
heparin	HEPARIN	
lepirudin	REFLUDAN	
reteplase	RETAVASE	
streptokinase	STREPTASE	KABIKINASE, STREPTASE
tenecteplase	TNKASE	
ticlopidine	TICLID	
tranexamic acid	CYKLOKAPRON, LYSTEDA	CYKLOKAPRON
urokinase – uPA	ABBOKINASE, KINLYTIC	ABBOKINASE
warfarin	COUMADIN, JANTOVEN	COUMADIN

Hemostasis and Erythropoiesis

Hemostasis Pathology and Pharmacotherapy

Pathologies associated with clotting failure can result from defects in thrombogenic proteins or platelet dysfunction. Most soluble clotting factors are synthesized in the liver. Therefore, liver disease or genetic mutations in clotting cascade proteins can result in bleeding diatheses. Similarly, dysfunction of platelets or decreased synthesis can result from genetic or secondary causes. Drugs in this chapter include:
1. Anticoagulants – Block clot formation by inhibiting the clotting cascade or platelet aggregation
2. Thrombolytics – Dissolve pathologic clots
3. Procoagulants – Enable clot formation

Clotting

Drugs that affect the clotting cascade can be used to prevent or to facilitate clotting. The processes regulating clot formation are extremely important in normal physiology because a clot can inhibit massive blood loss, but can also completely occlude blood flow to critical structures.

Pathological thrombi manifest in some very common clinical scenarios. Venous thrombi are associated with Virchow's triad:
1. Venous stasis
2. Vascular injury
3. Hypercoagulability

COMMON MANIFESTATIONS
- Pulmonary embolism → hypoxemia and right sided heart failure (if chronic)
- Deep venous thrombosis → pain, tenderness, edema in affected region
- Coronary plaque rupture → myocardial infarction (ST elevation)
- Ischemic stroke
  - Cerebrovascular occlusion usually resulting from embolus from heart or carotids
  - High risk conditions for cerebral embolus:
    - Atrial fibrillation
    - Valvular disease
    - Carotid plaque rupture or dislodgement

Hematopoietic Drugs

ERYTHROPOIETIN (rHuEPO)
MOA
- Erythropoietin receptor activation stimulates CFU (colony-forming unit) cells and to a lesser extent BFU (burst-forming unit) cells to promote proliferation, differentiation and survival (anti-apoptosis)
  - CFU and BFU are progenitor cells of RBCs

USES
- Anemia associated with:
  - Chronic renal disease
    - Administered 1-3 times per week
    - 2-6 weeks response lag
  - Cancer
  - HIV patients on **ZIDOVUDINE/AZIDOTHYMIDINE**

PK
- IV or subcutaneously
  - Subcutaneous → longer half-life (lower dose required)
- Intraperitoneal for dialysis patients

ADRs
- Primary hypertension, or worsening
- Increased risk of thrombotic events

NOTES
- Endogenous EPO is made in the kidney in response to hypoxia
- Acts in the marrow via JAK/STAT pathway
  - Found in greatest concentration on erythroid progenitor cells
- **DARBEPOETIN ALFA** is a more stable form with a longer half-life

Thrombolytics

Thrombolytics (Clot Busters)

MOA
- Convert or facilitate conversion of the inactive enzyme plasminogen into its active form
- Several drugs are classified as thrombolytics, each with similar mechanism of action but slightly different profiles
- These drugs directly or indirectly activate plasminogen

USES
- Early during thrombotic occlusion events
  - Coronary artery occlusion (within 4 hours)
  - Ischemic stroke (tPA within first 3 hours) – must rule out hemorrhage
  - Multiple pulmonary emboli

PK
- Short $t_{1/2}$ (30 minutes-1 hour)

ADRs
- Bleeding (cerebral hemorrhage = worst)
- Break down of physiological (good) clots
- Allergic response to STREPTOKINASE after multiple uses (foreign protein)

CONTRAINDICATIONS
- Active bleeding
- Surgery within past 10 days
- Serious GI bleeding within 3 months
- Severe hypertension
- Previous cerebral vascular accident (intracranial bleeding)

NOTES
- Directly acting enzymes
  - TISSUE PLASMINOGEN ACTIVATOR – tPA (human protein)
  - ALTEPLASE (recombinant human tPA)
  - RETEPLASE (recombinant human tPA)
  - TENECTEPLASE
  - UROKINASE- uPA (from human kidney)
- Indirectly acting – not enzymes
  - STREPTOKINASE (bacterial)
  - ANISTREPLASE (long-acting 1-2 hours)
- Plasmin is not given because it is inhibited by endogenous plasma anti-plasmins

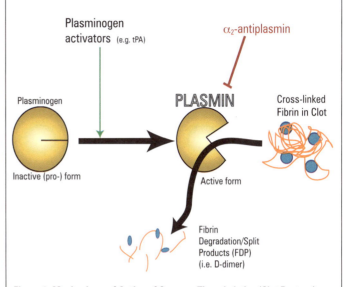

Figure 1. Mechanisms of Action of Common Thrombolytics (Clot Busters)

Hemostatics

TRANEXAMIC ACID

MOA
- Inhibits fibrinolysis by competitively blocking the binding of plasminogen to fibrin

USES
- Hemorrhage in hemophilia
- Menorrhagia

PK
- Short $t_{1/2}$ (2 hours)

ADRs
- Headache
- Sinus symptoms
- Back, abdominal, musculoskeletal pain
- Anemia
- Fatigue

AMINOCAPROIC ACID

MOA
- Inhibits fibrinolysis by competitively blocking the binding of plasminogen to fibrin

USES
- Antidote to thrombolytic overdose

PK
- Short $t_{1/2}$ (2 hours)

ADRs
- Nausea, vomiting
- Asthenia

CONTRAINDICATIONS
- Disseminated Intravascular Coagulation (DIC)
- Risk of thrombosis
- Premature neonates (injectable product contains benzyl alcohol)

Anticoagulants

HEPARIN

MOA

Unfractionated Heparin
- Binds to and amplifies the effect of antithrombin III (ATIII). ATIII inhibits factors Xa, IIa, and IXa
  - Prolongs partial thromboplastin time (PTT)
  - Acts on preformed components – instantaneous action both *in vitro* and *in vivo*

Low Molecular Weight Heparin (LMWH) = ENOXAPARIN
- LMWH has significant activity against factor Xa but less activity against thrombin (factor IIa) – no effect on PTT

USES
INPATIENT – short half life and administration route (parenteral)
- Immediate anticoagulation for suspected or confirmed:
  - Pulmonary embolism
  - Stroke
  - Angina
  - Myocardial infarction
  - DVT
  - Anticoagulation during pregnancy (since the drug does not cross the placenta)

PK
- Fast on/fast off – acts in blood
- Short $t_{1/2}$ (1.5 hours)
- LMWH – better bioavailability and longer half life, subcutaneous administration

ADRs
- Bleeding diathesis
- Heparin Induced Thrombocytopenia (HIT) – heparin forms immune complex with platelets and produces platelet thrombosis
- Osteoporosis with chronic use

CONTRAINDICATIONS
- Active bleeding
- Severe thrombocytopenia
- When blood coagulation tests cannot be performed at regular intervals (i.e. patients on this drug must be monitored closely)

NOTES
- Typically given parenterally

COUMARINS: WARFARIN

MOA
- Inhibits vitamin K dependent clotting factor synthesis (II, VII, IX, X, C, S) by blocking the enzyme vitamin K decarboxylase in the liver
- *In vivo* functionality only
- Prolongs PT and INR

USES
OUTPATIENT – long half-life and administration route (oral)
- Chronic anticoagulation

PK
- Long $t_{1/2}$ (1 week)
- Slow on/slow off

ADRs
- Warfarin skin necrosis (paradoxical clot resulting from lost protein C and S)
- Bleeding diathesis

CONTRAINDICATIONS
- Eclampsia
- Alcoholism
- Anaesthesia
- Aneurysms
- Endocarditis
- Hemorrhage
- Pericarditis
- Pregnancy (teratogenic)
- Surgery

DRUG INTERACTIONS
- Antibiotics
- Antifungals
- SSRIs
- Antiplatelet agents
- **AMIODARONE**
- **ACETAMINOPHEN**

NOTES
- Low therapeutic index, monitoring of INR required

Antidote to Heparin Overdose

PROTAMINE SULFATE
- **Positively charged protein from salmon sperm that binds to and rapidly reverses the effects of negatively charged heparin**

All anticoagulants can cause bleeding.

Antidotes to Warfarin Overdose

Vitamin K
- Slow acting (stimulates factor synthesis in liver)

Fresh Frozen Plasma (FFP)
- Fast acting (direct factor replacement)

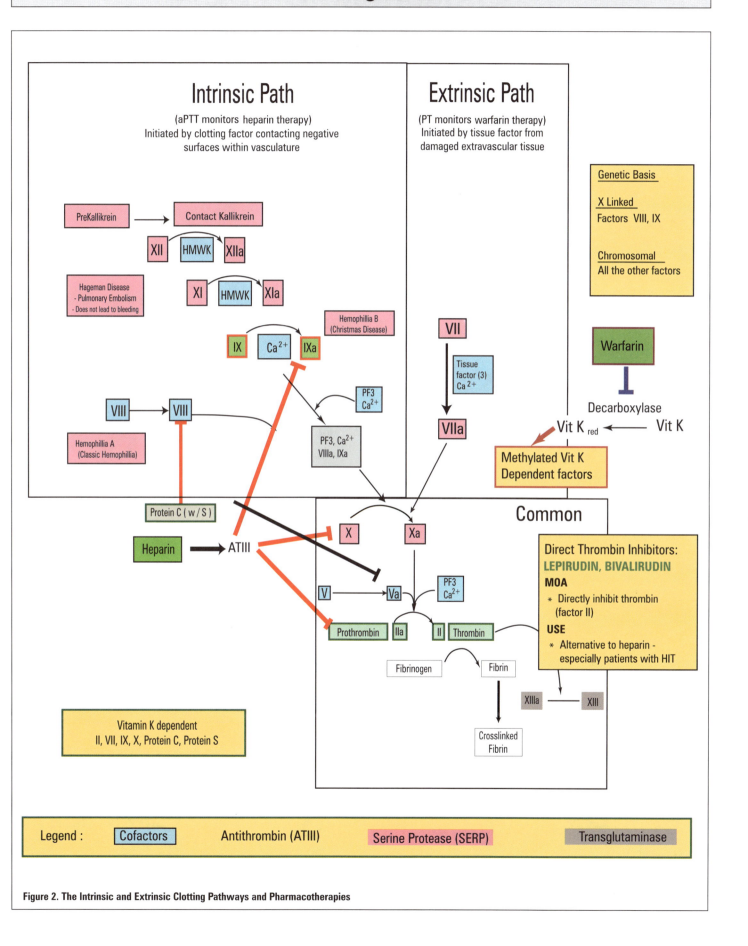

Figure 2. The Intrinsic and Extrinsic Clotting Pathways and Pharmacotherapies

Antiplatelet Drugs

PHYSIOLOGY OF PLATELET ACTIVATION
- Endothelial injury exposes subendothelial collagen to blood
- Platelets are activated by a number of factors
    - Collagen (via GP1a), serotonin, thrombin, epinephrine
    - Adenosine disphosphate (ADP)
    - Thromboxane A_2 (TXA_2) – created by COX enzymes from phospholipids in platelet membrane
- Activated platelets express activated GPIIb-IIIa on their surface
- The GPIIb-IIIa integrin receptor binds to and links platelets to fibrin strands in the growing clot
    - Under high flow conditions GPIIb-IIIa will also bind to vWF

There are three pharmacologically targeted sites in platelet activation:
1. ADP receptor
2. COX enzymes
3. GPIIb-IIIa

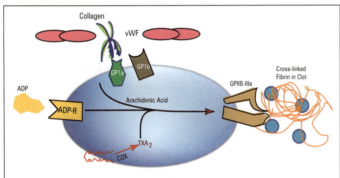

Figure 3. Physiology of Platelet Activation

ASPIRIN
MOA
- Irreversibly inhibits COX-1 and COX-2, decreases conversion of arachidonic acid to TXA_2, prevents expression of GPIIb-IIIa (effect: long BT, normal PTT, normal PT)

USES
- Antiplatelet (low dose)
    - **Primary preventative**
        - High risk patients >50 years of age for ischemic coronary artery disease or cerebral vascular disease
    - **Secondary preventative**
        - Previous MI, stroke or TIA, stable and unstable angina, severe carotid artery disease
- Antipyresis
- Analgesia (high dose for arthritis)
- Antiinflammatory

PK
- Short $t_{1/2}$ (15-20 minutes)
- Effects are long lasting because of irreversible inhibition of COX

ADRs
- Gastric ulcers
- Bleeding
- Hyperventilation (due to metabolic acidosis)
- Tinnitus
- Gout (low dose competes with uric acid for secretion)

CONTRAINDICATIONS
- Children and teenagers with chickenpox or flu-like symptoms (risk of Reye's syndrome)
- Syndrome of asthma, rhinitis, and nasal polyps

CLOPIDOGREL
MOA
- Prodrug activated by CYP2C19 in liver
- Irreversibly inhibits ADP receptor ($P2Y_{12}$) on platelets and consequently inhibits IIb/IIIa expression

USES
- **Secondary prevention**
- Ischemic CV disease, recent MI, recent thrombotic stroke
- Acute coronary syndrome
- Prevents thrombotic complications during percutaneous coronary intervention (PCI) and in particular stent replacement

PK
- Platelet aggregation returns to normal after 5 days
- Moderate $t_{1/2}$ (6 hours)

ADRs
- Bleeding
- Thrombotic Thrombocytopenic Purpura (TTP)
- Rare neutropenia (especially with **TICLOPIDINE**)

CONTRAINDICATIONS
- Active bleeding

NOTES
- Similar drugs: **TICLOPIDINE**

ABCIXIMAB
MOA
- Fab fragment of a monoclonal antibody directed against glycoprotein (GP) IIb-IIIa
- Sterically blocks platelet activation and aggregation

USES
- Percutaneous Coronary Interventions (PCI)
- Balloon angioplasty and stent placement

PK
- Normal platelet aggregation within 1 day of discontinuation
- Rapid elimination $t_{1/2}$ (30 minutes)

ADRs
- Very similar to **Unfractionated Heparin**
- Bleeding
- Thrombocytopenia

CONTRAINDICATIONS
- Bleeding diathesis
- History of vasculitis
- Intracranial tumor
- Major surgery (within 6 weeks)
- Uncontrolled hypertension
- Thrombocytopenia

Black Box Warning

CYP2C19 poor metabolizers cannot form active metabolite as efficiently, therefore higher cardiovascular event rates are seen in patients treated for acute coronary sydrome or PCI with **CLOPIDOGREL** at recommended doses.

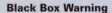

Immune Response Modifiers

Chapter Authors: Nicholas D. Boespflug, Andrew W. Browne, Violette M.G.J. Gijsen and Norris I. Hollie

Faculty Reviewers: Amit Govil, Nicole M. Schmidt and John W. Semple

IN THIS CHAPTER

Immune Modulators	132
Immunosuppressors	133
Immunoenhancers	136
Dermatologic Drugs	138
Gout	140

DRUGS IN THIS CHAPTER

Generic Name	US Trade Name	Canadian Trade Name
acitretin	SORIATANE	
adalimumab	HUMIRA	
aldesleukin	PROLEUKIN	
alemtuzumab	CAMPATH	MABCAMPATH
allopurinol	ZYLOPRIM	ALLOPURINOL, ZYLOPRIM ALLOPRIN
azathioprine	AZASAN, IMURAN	IMURAN
basiliximab	SIMULECT	
BCG vaccine	THERACYS, TICE BCG	IMMUCYST
colchicine	COLSALIDE, COLCRYS	
cyclophosphamide	CYTOXAN	CYTOXAN, PROCYTOX
cyclosporine A	RESTASIS, SANDIMMUNE	NEORAL, SANDIMMUNE
daclizumab	ZENAPAX	
darbepoetin Alfa	ARANESP	
etanercept	ENBREL	
filgrastim	NEUPOGEN	
finasteride	PROPECIA, PROSCAR	
human IgG (IVIG)	FLEBOGAMMA, OCTAGAM, GAMMAGARD, GAMUNEX, CARIMUNE	GAMASTAN, GAMMAGARD, GAMUNEX, PRIVIGEN, SANDOGLOBULIN
indomethacin	INDOCIN	NU-INDO
infliximab	REMICADE	
isotretinoin	ACCUTANE, AMNESTEEM, CLARAVIS, SOTRET	ACCUTANE, CLARUS
minoxidil	LONITEN, ROGAINE	LONITEN, ROGAINE, APOGAIN
muromonab-CD3	ORTHOCLONE OKT3	
mycophenolate mofetil	CELLCEPT	
prednisone	DELTASONE, PREDNICOT, PREDNISONE INTENSOL, STERAPRED	DELTASONE, WINPRED
probenecid	BENEMID, PROBALAN	BENEMID, BENURYL
recombinant interferon-alpha	INFERGEN	INTRON A
rho (D) immune globulin	BAYRHO-D, WINRHO SDF, MICRHOGAM, RHOGAM, RHOPHYLAC, HYPERRHO	WINRHO SDF
RIFN-β	AVONEX, REBIF	AVONEX, BETASERON, REBIF
RIFN-γ	ACTIMMUNE	
rituximab	RITUXAN	
sargramostim	LEUKINE	
sirolimus	RAPAMUNE	
tacrolimus	PROGRAF, PROTOPIC	ADVAGRAF, PROGRAF, PROTOPIC
thalidomide	THALOMID	
thymalfasin	ZADAXIN	

Immune Modulators

Pharmacotherapy is used to alter the immune system when it is unable to clear the offending agent (cancer, infection) or because it has been inappropriately activated towards endogenous or innocuous agents (arthritis, lupus, allergy). For specific clinical scenarios where immunomodulation is desired, it is important to recognize the components of an immune response that are active (or inactive) so that the correct therapy may be employed.

Antibodies have become important pharmacologic immunomodulators. Immune cells sense the extracellular environment and the status of neighboring cells by recognizing proteins (antigens) bound to surface receptors. In the case of an overactive immune response, antibodies can be used as therapy that bind to these surface receptors and effectively blind the immune system.

Unfortunately, exogenous antibodies are foreign proteins and can elicit anaphylaxis or other hypersensitivity reactions in the recipient.

The following pages contain drugs that modulate the immune response at a specific stage. For immunomodulators, the reaction is broken into antigen presentation, T-cell recognition and immune response by effector cells. Many drugs work at the T-cell recognition stage. Some are antibodies that block the interaction of T-cells with antigen presenting cells (APCs). Some antibodies block receptors on T-cells so they are unable to receive survival and effector cytokine signals (**BASILIXIMAB**, and the anti-TNF antibodies). The calcineurin inhibitors (**TACROLIMUS**, **CYCLOSPORIN A**) interfere with the intracellular signaling cascades that occur as a T-cell becomes activated and culminate in transcription factor activation. The effector stage of the immune reaction can be modulated by antibodies that target certain subsets of immune cells for destruction (**ALEMTUZUMAB**, **RITUXUMAB**) or by the use of cytotoxic drugs (akin to chemotherapeutics) that target rapidly dividing cells (a critical feature of immune responses) by damaging DNA or inhibiting DNA synthesis.

The immunostimulators are presented similarly with the added stages of hematopoiesis occurring before the rest of the immune response. Here, drugs are employed to increase the numbers of important precursor cells (**FILGRASTIM**, **SARGRAMOSTIM** and **RHEPO**), stimulate immune cells to proliferate (**ALDESLEUKIN**, **THYMOSIN**), replace natural antibodies (human IgG) or increase effector function (**BCG**, **INTERFERON**, **THALIDOMIDE**).

Hypersensitivities

Five different types of hypersensitivity reaction can occur:
- Type I – Immediate hypersensitivity (mast cell degranulation; can result in anaphylactic shock)
- Type II – Cytotoxic hypersensitivity (antibodies bind antigen on the patient's own cells)
- Type III – Immune complex disease (antigen-antibody complexes that can lodge in kidneys or cause vasculitis)
- Type IV – Delayed type hypersensitivty (cell-mediated reaction, antibody independent)
- Type V – Autoimmune disease

Transplant

Transplants require immunomodulation due to two broad immune reactions, both of which require therapy that decreases the immune response:

Transplant Rejection
- The recipient attacks the transplant
- Hyperacute – complement mediated due to preexisting antibodies to the donor (mismatched ABO blood type), almost immediate effects
- Acute – T-cell mediated, onset approximately a few days after transplantation
- Chronic – less well understood recurrent inflammation of transplant

Graft versus Host Disease (GvHD)
- The marrow/blood transplant attacks the recipient

Immunosuppressive drugs are given at specific stages during the transplantation process. The transplant recipient must be immunosuppressed before receiving the transplant (INDUCTION). Immunosuppression must be maintained after transplant to prevent rejection (MAINTENANCE). Other agents must be used to treat REJECTION or GvHD, if these develop.

Suppressing the immune system causes adverse effects. Perhaps the most obvious is susceptibility to infections, especially latent fungal or viral pathogens. Another more immediate adverse effect is due to the nature of immune cells. Activated T-lymphocytes can secrete cytokines to amplify and regulate the immune response. When antibodies bind to a T-cell, it releases cytokines resulting in a systemic inflammatory reaction. This results in cytokine release syndrome which can can result in flu-like symptoms or general malaise.

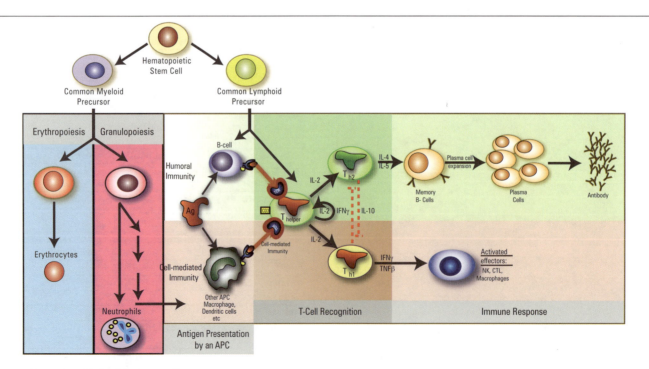

Figure 1. Generation of Cells of the Immune Response

Immunosuppressors

Antiproliferative Drugs

SIROLIMUS

MOA
- Binds to FK506-binding protein-12 (FKBP12) which then binds to and inhibits the mammalian Target of Rapamycin (mTOR)
- Inhibits cell cycle progression
- Inhibits interleukin (IL)-2, 4, and 15

USES
- Cardiac, islet cell, kidney, liver, lung: immunosuppression, rejection, GvHD
- Thrombotic microangiopathy

PK
- Very long $t_{1/2}$ (57-63 hours)

ADRs
- Hypercholesterolemia
- Hyperlipidemia
- Hypertriglyceridemia
- Impaired wound healing
- Proteinuria
- Inhibition of CYP3A4
- Thrombocytopenia

DRUG INTERACTIONS
- **CYCLOSPORINE** increases the bioavailability of sirolimus – synergy – **SIROLIMUS** should be taken 4 hours after **CYCLOSPORINE**
- Concomitant use of **TACROLIMUS** and **SIROLIMUS** may result in decreased levels of **TACROLIMUS** – close monitoring is recommended
- Inhibitors and inducers of CYP3A4 can alter the systemic exposure – monitor closely

Calcineurin Inhibitors

CYCLOSPORINE A (CsA)

MOA
- Binds to cyclophillin which then binds to calcineurin to inhibit T-cell activation

USES
- Certain autoimmune diseases: rheumatoid arthritis, psoriasis, uveitis, immune thrombocytopenia (ITP)
- AIDS
- Certain muscle diseases: amyotrophic lateral sclerosis (ALS), Duchenne muscular dystrophy (DMD)
- Transplant: immunosuppression, rejection, GvHD

PK
- Long $t_{1/2}$ (19 hours)

ADRs
- Nephrotoxicity (more often than **TACROLIMUS**)
- Neurotoxicity (less often than **TACROLIMUS**)
- Hirsutism
- Hypertension
- Hyperlipidemia

DRUG INTERACTIONS
- Synergistic with **TACROLIMUS**

TACROLIMUS

MOA
- Inhibits T-lymphocyte activation by binding to FKBP which inhibits calcineurin phosphatase

USES
- Transplant: immunosuppression, GvHD
- Certain autoimmune diseases: rheumatoid arthritis, psoriasis, uveitis

PK
- Moderate $t_{1/2}$ (11 hours)

ADRs
- Diabetes Mellitus
- Insomnia
- Alopecia
- Hypertension
- Hypomagnesemia
- Nephrotoxicity
- Neurotoxicity
- Hyperkalemia

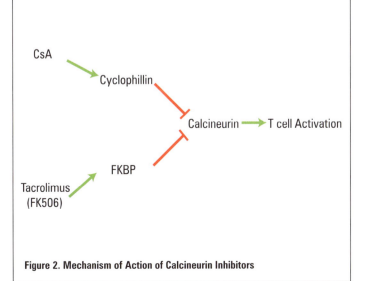

Figure 2. Mechanism of Action of Calcineurin Inhibitors

Immunosuppressors

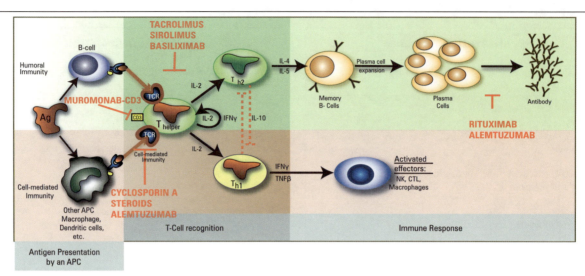

Figure 3. Cells of the Immune Response

Steroids

PREDNISONE (Corticosteroid)

MOA
- Works through corticosteroid binding globulin
  - Binds cytoplasmic receptor/Hsp90
  - Hsp90 dissociates and translocates to nucleus
1. Block cytokine production
2. Block T-cell proliferation → rapid, transient reduction in peripheral blood lymphocytes (T and B)

USES
- Transplant: immunosuppression, rejection, GvHD
- Autoimmune disease
- Asthma
- Myasthenia gravis, DMD, myositis, acute MS, temporal arteritis, cluster headache

PK
- Short $t_{1/2}$ (2-3 hours)

ADRs
- Shut down HPA (Hypothalamic-Pituitary-Adrenal Axis)
- Fluid abnormalilites (salt retention)
- Osteoporosis
- Cataracts
- Growth arrest
- Muscle wasting
- Psychosis
- Diabetes (hyperglycemia)
- Adrenal insufficiency symptoms
- Inhaled preparations → thrush, vocal hoarseness

NOTES
- Withdrawal of steroids must be done slowly to allow for the adrenal gland to recommence endogenous production

Cytotoxic Compounds

CYCLOPHOSPHAMIDE

MOA
- Covalently alkylates DNA → mispairs, crosslinks
  - Cytotoxic to proliferating lymphocytes (T < B)
  - Blocks ongoing immune reactions
  - Similar action in proliferating cancer cells

USES
- Transplant: immunosuppression in certain types of transplant
- Autoimmune diseases: rheumatoid arthritis, Sjögren's syndrome, systemic lupus erythematosus

OTHER INFORMATION
- see Cancer Chemotherapeutics chapter

AZATHIOPRINE

MOA
- Prodrug that is rapidly metabolized to **6-MERCAPTOPURINE**
- Immunosuppressive antimetabolite

USES
- Kidney, liver, pancreas transplant
- Autoimmune diseases: rheumatoid arthritis, ankylosing spondylitis, systemic lupus erythematosus, myasthenia gravis
- Atopic dermatitis

OTHER INFORMATION
- See **6-MERCAPTOPURINE** in the Cancer Chemotherapeutics chapter

MYCOPHENOLATE MOFETIL/MYCOPHENOLIC ACID

MOA
- Inhibits inosine monophosphate dehydrogenase and blocks purine synthesis, leading to inhibition of lymphocyte proliferation

USES
- Cardiac, kidney, liver transplant: immunosuppression, rejection, GvHD
- Autoimmune diseases
  - Myasthenia gravis, thrombocytopenia, psoriasis, rheumatoid arthritis, systemic lupus erythematosus

PK
- Moderate to long $t_{1/2}$ (8-18 hours)

ADRs
- **GI distress**
- **Leukopenia**
- Hypertension
- Peripheral edema
- Hypercholesterolemia
- Hyperglycemia
- Electrolyte imbalance
- Hemorrhagic cystitis (**CYCLOPHOSPHAMIDE**)

Immunosuppressors

Biologics (Antibodies)

ETANERCEPT, INFLIXIMAB, ADALIMUMAB
MOA
- Binds to TNFα and renders it biologically inactive

USES
- Autoimmune diseases
  - Crohn's disease
  - Rheumatoid arthritis – slow acting anti-rheumatic drug (SAARD)
  - Ankylosing spondylitis
  - Psoriasis
  - GvHD

PK
- Very long $t_{1/2}$ (days)

ADRs
- Upper respiratory infection
- Rhinitis
- Neutropenic disorder
- Leukopenia

RITUXIMAB
MOA
- Murine/human monoclonal antibody that binds to the CD20 antigen and mediates B-cell lysis and destruction

USES
- Autoimmune diseases: hemolytic anemia, rheumatoid arthritis, systemic lupus erythematosus, Evans syndrome, pemphigus vulgaris, ITP
- Oncology: B-cell lymphoma, chronic lymphoid leukemia, hairy cell leukemia, Hodgkin's disease, CD20-positive non-Hodgkin's lymphoma, Waldenström macroglobulinemia
- Transplant: GvHD, post-transplant lymphoproliferative disorder
- Thrombocytopenic purpura
- Wegener's granulomatosis

PK
- Very long $t_{1/2}$ (days)

ADRs
- Cardiovascular: hypertension and hypotension, dysrhythmia, cardiogenic shock, arrhythmia
- Neurological: asthenia, sensory neuropathy
- Hematologic: cytopenia

NOTES
- Fatal infusion reactions may occur within 24 hours of RITUXIMAB infusion; approximately 80% of fatal reactions occur with first infusion

ALEMTUZUMAB
MOA
- Humanized monoclonal antibody against CD52 cell surface glycoproteins
- Binds to B-cells and T-cells and induces cell lysis

USES
- Autoimmune disease: rheumatoid arthritis, celiac disease
- Oncology: B-cell chronic lymphocytic leukemia, primary cutaneous T-cell lymphoma, T-cell prolymphocytic leukemia
- Transplant: hemopoietic stem cell transplant, renal transplantation
- Relapsing remitting multiple sclerosis
- Vasculitis

PK
- Very long $t_{1/2}$ (12 days)

ADRs
- Hematologic: anemia, neutropenia, thrombocytopenia
- Infusion reaction

MUROMONAB-CD3
MOA
- Binds to CD3 antigen on T-cell surface. This inactivates the T-cell receptor, which prevents activation of the T-lymphocyte

USES
- Cardiac, kidney, liver, lung transplant: immunosuppression, rejection, GvHD
- T-cell acute lymphoblastic leukemia
- Lymphocytic myocarditis
- Psoriasis vulgaris

PK
- Long $t_{1/2}$ (18 hours)

ADRs
- Hypertension, hypotension, tachycardia
- Encephalopathy
- Cytokine release syndrome

Rho(D) IMMUNE GLOBULIN
MOA
- Human IgG that binds and blocks maternal antibodies from eliciting an immune response to fetal blood

USES
- Given to Rh(-) mothers with a possibility of a Rh(+) pregnancy
- Hemolytic disease of the newborn
- Prior Rh(+) birth in an Rh(-) mom with rising titers
- Immune thrombocytopenia purpura (in Rh(+) patients with an intact spleen)

PK
- Very long $t_{1/2}$ (24-30 days)

ADRs
- Extravascular hemolysis

BASILIXIMAB (IL-2 receptor antagonists)
MOA
- Binds to the IL-2 receptor and inhibits IL-2 binding and therefore activation of lymphocytes

USES
- Transplant: cardiac, liver, kidney and pancreas transplantation, GvHD
- Psoriasis
- Aplastic anemia
- Acquired epidermolysis bullosa

PK
- Very long $t_{1/2}$ (7 days)

ANTITHYMOCYTE GLOBULIN (ATG)
MOA
- Binds to thymocytes (T-cells); inhibits their activation and mediates their lysis and destruction

USES
- Transplant: treatment of acute rejection in renal transplant

PK
- Very long $t_{1/2}$ (2-3 days)

ADRs
- Cytokine release syndrome

Immunosuppressants and Live Vaccines

An inadequate immunological reaction response to the vaccine may occur.
The concomitant use should be avoided and patients should be advised that the vaccines may be less effective.

Immunoenhancers

Immune Serum

HUMAN IgG (IVIG)

MOA
- Mechanism is unclear but believed to block Fc receptors thereby inhibiting macrophage and dendritic cell activation
- Reduces the production or blocks the activity of IL-1
- Net effect is to suppress inflammation

USES
- Primary immunodeficiencies
- Chronic inflammatory demyelinating polyneuropathy (CIDP)
- Bone marrow transplant
- Kawasaki disease
- Chronic lymphocytic leukemia
- Transplant: rejection
- ITP

PK
- Very long $t_{1/2}$ (3-6 weeks)

ADRs
- Headache
- Injection site reaction
- Arthralgia
- Pain in limb
- Flushing
- Chills
- Nausea
- Acute renal failure
- Thrombotic complications

T-cell Stimulators

ALDESLEUKIN

MOA
- Induction of cytotoxic T-cells
- Enhancement lymphocyte mitogenesis

USES
- Melanoma
- Renal cell carcinoma
- Acute myeloid leukemia
- Epstein-Barr virus disease

PK
- Short $t_{1/2}$ (85 minutes)

ADRs
- Hypotension
- Loss of appetite
- Stomatitis

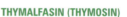

THYMALFASIN (THYMOSIN)

MOA
- Stimulates T-cell maturation in thymus

USES
- Hepatitis C
- Hepatitis D
- HIV infection
- Malignant melanoma
- Non-small cell lung cancer
- Di George syndrome

DARBEPOETIN ALFA

MOA
- Recombinant erythropoietin
- Stimulates the production and differentiation of red blood cells

USES
- Anemia due to chemotherapy
- Anemia of chronic kidney disease

PK
- Very long $t_{1/2}$ (46-74 hours)

ADRs
- Edema
- Hypotension
- Hypertension
- Upper respiratory infections

BACILLUS OF CALMETTE AND GUERIN (BCG) VACCINE

MOA
- Live vaccine from a strain of *Mycobacterium bovis*
- Mechanism largely unknown
  - Oncology: live bacteria may provoke a local immune response that clears tumor
  - Autoimmune: live bacteria may divert the immune response from autoimmune reaction to clear the infection

USES
- Oncology: tumors of the bladder, leukemia, colon cancer, breast cancer
- Tuberculosis vaccination
- Multiple sclerosis

ADRs
- Dysuria
- Urinary frequency
- Hematuria
- Cystitis

NOTES
- False positive for tests of tuberculosis

Immunoenhancers

Colony Stimulating Factor

FILGRASTIM
MOA
- Human granulocyte-colony stimulating factor (G-CSF)
- Stimulates neutrophil and progenitor cells production and differentiation

USES
- Neutropenia
- Neutropenic disorder
- Harvesting of peripheral blood stem cells
- Leukemia

PK
- Short $t_{1/2}$ (3.5 hours)

ADRs
- Bone pain

SARGRAMOSTIM
MOA
- Human granulocyte-macrophage colony-stimulating factor (GM-CSF)
- Stimulates proliferation and differentiation of neutrophils, progenitor cells, myeloid-derived dendritic cells, and monocytes/macrophages

USES
- Bone marrow transplantation
- Neutropenia
- Harvesting of peripheral blood stem cells
- Peripheral blood stem cell allograft

PK
- Short $t_{1/2}$ (60-162 minutes)

ADRs
- Chest pain
- Increased bilirubin level
- Asthenia
- Fever
- Metabolic disease
- Arthralgia

Effector Stimulators

RECOMBINANT INTERFERON-α (RIFN-α2A and RIFN-α2B)
MOA
- Type I interferon
- Stimulate macrophages and NK cells to elicit an antiviral response

USES
- Chronic myeloid leukemia
- Chronic hepatitis C
- Hairy cell leukemia

PK
- Moderate $t_{1/2}$ (4-8.5 hours)

ADRs
- Alopecia
- Taste alterations, anorexia
- GI disorders
- Neutropenia
- Depression
- Hypocalcemia, hypophosphatemia

RIFN-β
MOA
- Type I interferon
- Similar to IFN-α

USES
- Multiple sclerosis

PK
- Moderate $t_{1/2}$ (4-10 hours)

ADRs
- Decreased lymphocyte count
- Increased muscle tone
- Myalgia
- Asthenia
- Depression
- Influenza-like symptoms

RIFN-γ
MOA
- Type II interferon
- Activates macrophages and increases lysosome activity in macrophages

USES
- Chronic granulomatous disease
- Malignant osteopetrosis

PK
- Short to moderate $t_{1/2}$ (2-8 hours)

ADRs
- Influenza-like symptoms

THALIDOMIDE
MOA
- Unknown

USES
- Erythema nodosum leprosum
- Multiple myeloma

PK
- Moderate $t_{1/2}$ (5-7 hours)

ADRs
- Peripheral neuropathy
- Deep vein thrombosis

Dermatologic Drugs

Dermatological drugs focus on treatments for severe acne, hair loss and skin inflammation.

Corticosteroids are commonly used to minimize inflammation. They are permeable through the cell membrane and bind to specific receptors in the nucleus to affect gene transcription. Topical corticosteroids are divided into seven classes based on efficacy, of which only classes 4 and 5 are used by dermatologists. They have many adverse effects and are used prudently.

Derivatives of vitamin A are used to treat severe acne. Though highly effective for acne vulgaris and psoriasis, they carry many severe adverse effects. Derivatives of vitamin A are severe teratogens, and women are required to be on two forms of birth control while on the drug. In addition, severe liver damage can lead to dangerously high triglyceride levels.

Trichogenic agents, such as **FINASTERIDE** and **MINOXIDIL**, support hair growth via different mechanisms and have very different adverse effect profiles.

DERMATOLOGICAL THERAPIES
- Drug + Vehicle to deliver the drug

CHOICE OF VEHICLE IS VERY IMPORTANT
- If the skin is dry → use a moistening vehicle
- If the skin is wet → use a drying vehicle

Vehicle	Wetting/Drying	Comments
Tincture	Most drying	Alcohol-based
Shake Lotion	Drying	Water-based
Solution	Drying	
Cream	Wetting	
Ointment	Wetting	Greasy (most common vehicle)
Oils	Most wetting	

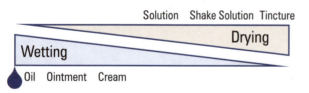

Topical Corticosteroids

The basis of classification of relative corticosteroid efficacy is based on their ability to cause vasoconstriction (NOT their anti-inflammatory properties).
- Vasoconstriction is the desired effect in topically applied steroids

Class	Potency	Examples
Class 1	Extremely potent	**CLOBETASOL**
Class 2 + 3	Potent	**FLUCINONIDE**
Class 4 + 5	Intermediate	**BETAMETHASONE VALERATE**
Class 6 + 7	Mild	**HYDROCORTISONE**

Class 4 and 5
Topical Corticosteroids

USES
- Anti-inflammatory – relief of inflammatory pruritus

MOA
- Vasoconstriction

ADRs
- High "potency" (efficacy) steroids should be avoided in intertriginous areas because they can cause skin thinning, atrophy, even ulceration
- Use with caution in children because absorption is greater and may cause skin atrophy and adrenal suppression (blunted HPA axis)

Dermatologic Drugs

Retinoids

ISOTRETINOIN

MOA
- Synthetic analogue of vitamin A
- Decreases the production of sebum

USES
- Nodulocystic acne (especially when scarring occurs)

PK
- Long $t_{1/2}$ (10-20 hours)

ADRs
- Dry skin
- Pruritus
- Retinoid dermatitis
- Abnormal lipids
- Raised erythrocyte sedimentation rate
- Conjunctivitis

ACITRETIN

MOA
- Unknown, but decreases inflammation and proliferation

USES
- Psoriasis

PK
- Very long $t_{1/2}$ (50 hours)

ADRs
- Alopecia
- Dry skin, dry mucous membranes
- Pancreatitis
- Night blindness

NOTES
- Both **ISOTRETINOIN** and **ACITRETIN** are teratogenic – cannot be used in pregnancy or those seeking to become pregnant

Trichogenic (Hair Growth) Agents

FINASTERIDE

MOA
- Inhibitor of the enzyme 5α-reductase thereby preventing production of dihydroxytestosterone (DHT)

USES
- Hair growth
- Benign prostatic hyperplasia

PK
- Short to long $t_{1/2}$ (3-16 hours)

ADRs
- Rash
- Gynecomastia
- Diarrhea

MINOXIDIL

MOA
- K^+ channel activation → blood vessel dilation → stimulates vertex hair growth
- Selective vasodilatation of the arteriolar vessels

USES
- Refractory hypertension
- Male pattern alopecia in males and females

PK
- Moderate $t_{1/2}$ (4.2 hours)

Gout

The nephron is capable of passive filtration, reabsorption and active secretion of blood constituents. The proximal convoluted tubule is responsible for the active secretion of those blood constituents that were not filtered by the glomerulus. One of the most important classes of blood constituents that are actively secreted are the weak organic acids.

The following are the most pharmacologically and physiologically relevant weak organic acids that are actively secreted:
1. Water soluble vitamins:
   - Ascorbic acid (vitamin C)
   - Nicotinic acid (vitamin B3)
   - Folic acid
   - Pyradoxine (vitamin B6)
2. Drugs:
   - Penicillins
   - Cephalosporins
   - NSAIDs (e.g. aspirin)
   - Probenecid
3. Normal physiological components:
   - Uric acid

Secretion and reabsorption are saturable processes. When uric acid (i.e. urate) from the blood accumulates in the tissues, inflammation occurs. The signs and symptoms accompanying this inflammation are called gout. The basic pathophysiology of gout is:

↑ production or ↓ secretion of urate → hyperuricemia → precipitation, crystallization → inflammation (gout)

Treatment approaches include reducing production of urate (by inhibiting xanthine oxidase [XO]), stimulating urate excretion (by reducing reabsorption), and reducing inflammation from urate precipitation. Remember that:

(Filtration + Secretion) − Reabsorption = Excretion

Other Causes of Gout
- Leukemia/lymphoma
- Von Gierke's disease
- Furosemide and thiazides
- Lesch-Nyhan syndrome (hypoxanthine-guanine phosphoribosyltransferase deficiency shifts nucleic acids to XO pathway)
- Phosphoribosyl pyrophosphate excess leads to purine excess

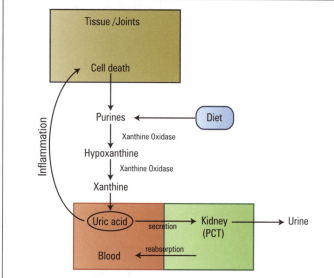

Figure 4. Pathophysiology of Gout

Prophylaxis

ALLOPURINOL
MOA
- Inhibits xanthine oxidase
- Increases reutilization of hypoxanthine and xanthine
- Decreases uric acid concentrations in serum and urine

USES
- Calcium renal calculus
- Hyperuricemia
- Gout
- During treatment for leukemia

PK
- Short $t_{1/2}$ (1-3 hours)

ADRs
- Maculopapular eruption
- Hepatotoxicity
- Pruritus

PROBENECID
MOA
- Low doses, inhibits the renal organic acid secretion (bad for gout)
- High doses, compete with and inhibits the reabsorption of uric acid in the proximal convoluted tubule
  - NET INCREASED EXCRETION

USES
- Adjunct to antibiotic therapy (prevents secretion of antibiotics)
- Gonorrhea (with **PENICILLIN** or **AMPICILLIN**)
- Hyperuricemia

PK
- Moderate $t_{1/2}$ (3-8 hours)

ADRs
- Anorexia
- Vomiting
- Rash
- Acute gout
- Nephrotoxic
- Allergic dermatitis

Acute Gout Therapy

COLCHICINE
MOA
- Binds to tubulin and inhibits microtubule assembly, thus preventing leukocyte migration, phagocytosis, and degranulation
- Inhibits the inflammatory response to urate crystals

USES
- Gout
- Familial Mediterranean fever

PK
- Very long $t_{1/2}$ (27-31 hours)

ADRs
- Diarrhea
- Nausea, vomiting

NOTES
- Has a low therapeutic index

INDOMETHACIN
MOA
- NSAID – reversibly inhibits COX-1 and COX-2

USES
- Ankylosing spondylitis
- Acute gout
- Osteoarthritis
- Acute pain
- Rheumatoid arthritis
- Patent ductus arteriosus

PK
- Moderate $t_{1/2}$ (4.5 hours)

ADRs
- Indigestion
- Tinnitus
- Depression

Renal and Urological Drugs

Chapter Authors: Andrew W. Browne, Patrina Gunness, Goutham Vemana and Paul Wiseman

Faculty Reviewer: Cindy Woodland

IN THIS CHAPTER

Urinary Continence and Incontinence................................	142
Renin-Angiotensin-Aldosterone System............................	144
Diuretics...	146
Carbonic Anhydrase Inhibitors (CAIs)	
Loop Diuretics	
Thiazide Diuretics	
Potassium-Sparing Diuretics	
Osmotic Diuretics	
Erectile Dysfunction..	152

DRUGS IN THIS CHAPTER

Generic Name	US Trade Name	Canadian Trade Name
acetazolamide	DIAMOX SEQUEL	
aliskiren	TEKTURNA	RASILEZ
amiloride	MIDAMOR	
bethanecol	URECHOLINE	DUVOID
captopril	CAPOTEN	
desmopressin	DDAVP, MINIRIN, STIMATE	DDAVP, MINIRIN, OCTOSTIM
doxazosin	CARDURA	
ethacrynic acid	EDECRIN	
finasteride	PROPECIA, PROSCAR	
furosemide	LASIX, FUROCOT, FUROMIDE M.D.	LASIX
hydrochlorothiazide	AQUAZIDE H, HYDROCOT, MICROZIDE, ZIDE	ACCURETIC, ALDACTAZIDE, ALTACE, ATACAND, AVALIDE, DIOVAN, HYZAAR, MICARDIS, RINZIDE, RASILEZ, TEVETEN, VASERETIC, VISKAZIDE, ZESTORETIC
imipramine	TOFRANIL	
lisinopril	PRINIVIL, ZESTRA	
losartan	COZAAR	
mannitol	OSMITROL, RESECTISOL	OSMITROL
oxybutynin	OXYTROL	
prazosin	MINIPRESS	
propantheline	PRO-BANTHINE	
sildenafil	REVATIO, VIAGRA	
spironolactone	ALDACTONE	
tadalafil	ADCIRCA, CIALIS	
tamsulosin	FLOMAX	
tolterodine	DETROL	
tolvaptan	SAMSCA	
torsemide	DEMADEX	
triamterene	DYRENIUM	
vardenafil	LEVITRA	

Urinary Continence and Incontinence

Bladder Function

The bladder is innervated by three sets of nerves

1. Sympathetic Nerves
- Activation of these nerves relaxes the bladder detrusor muscle and contracts the bladder outlet and urethra

2. Parasympathetic Nerves
- Activation of these nerves contracts the bladder and relaxes the urethral internal sphincter

3. Somatic Nerves
- Activation of these nerves results in the voluntary function of the external urethral sphincter

Urinary Bladder Mechanisms
β-adrenergic receptors
- Stimulation of β_2 and β_3-adrenoreceptors of the detrusor muscle results in the direct relaxation of the smooth muscle
- β-adrenergic receptor modulation, however, is not efficacious for treatment of bladder or urethral disorders

α-adrenergic receptors
- Stimulation of α-adrenoreceptors is not prominent in the normal bladder
- In pathological conditions, such as bladder overactivity and bladder outlet obstruction, research studies have found increased presence of these receptors (specifically α_{1D}-adrenoreceptors)
- The increased density of these α-adrenoreceptors can alter the response to NE from relaxation to contraction
- α-adrenergic mechanisms are more important in urethral function
- Urethral tone and intra-urethral pressure are significantly influenced by the activation of α-adrenoreceptors
- Inhibition of α-adrenoreceptors (specifically α_1-adrenoreceptors) facilitates bladder voiding by decreasing urethral resistance from a condition such as benign prostatic hyperplasia

Tricyclic Antidepressant (TCA)

IMIPRAMINE
MOA
- Blocks the uptake of NE and other neurotransmitters at nerve endings
- The exact mechanism of action of nocturnal enuresis is not fully elucidated but is largely related to the antimuscarinic effects of TCAs

USES
- Mood disorders (see CNS Drugs chapter)
- Nocturnal enuresis
- Urinary incontinence

PK
- Moderate to long $t_{1/2}$ (6-18 hours)

ADRs
- Antimuscarinic effects (dry mouth, urinary retention, constipation)
- Cardiovascular effects (orthostatic hypotension, tachycardia, hypertension, arrhythmias, T-wave abnormalities)
  - Dose-dependent cardiotoxicity
- CNS effects (sedation, decreased seizure threshold, delirium, confusion)
  - May precipitate manic episode in bipolar patients

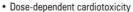
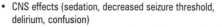

NOTES
- See CNS Drugs chapter for more information and additional TCAs

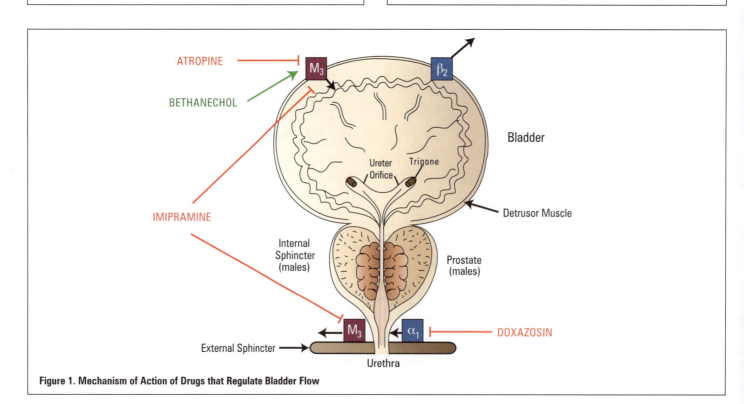

Figure 1. Mechanism of Action of Drugs that Regulate Bladder Flow

Urinary Continence and Incontinence

Medications that Stop Flow

Muscarinic Receptor Antagonists

OXYBUTYNIN, PROPANTHELINE, TOLTERODINE

MOA
- Muscarinic receptor antagonist → relaxation of smooth muscle

USES
- Overactive bladder
- Neurogenic bladder
- Urinary incontinence

PK OXYBUTYNIN
- Short $t_{1/2}$ (2-8 hours)

PK PROPANTHELINE
- Short $t_{1/2}$ (1.6 hours)

PK TOLTERODINE
- Variable

ADRs
- Constipation
- Angioedema
- Dry mouth
- Confusion
- Decreased sweating

CONTRAINDICATIONS
- Closed-angle glaucoma

Medications that Allow Flow

Muscarinic Receptor Agonist

BETHANECHOL

MOA
- Stimulates the release of ACh → increased tone of detrusor urinae muscle → initiation of micturation and bladder emptying

USES
- Urinary retention

ADRs
- **BLUSHPADS BBC**
  - **B**radycardia
  - **L**acrimation
  - **U**rination
  - **S**alivation
  - **H**ypotension
  - **P**inpoint Pupils (miosis)
  - **A**ccommodation
  - **D**efecation (increased GI motility)
  - **S**weating
  - **B**ronchoconstriction
  - **B**ronchosecretion
  - **C**NS dysfunction (ataxia, confusion)

CONTRAINDICATIONS
- Coronary artery disease
- Epilepsy
- Bronchial asthma
- Parkinsonism
- Severe bradycardia or hypotension
- Strength or integrity of the GI or bladder wall is uncertain
- GI obstruction
- Vasomotor instability

Type II 5α Reductase Inhibitor

FINASTERIDE

MOA
- Competitive blockade of 5α reductase, an enzyme involved in the synthesis of dihydroxytestosterone (DHT)
- Reverses androgen DHT-dependent prostate gland development (effect requires months)

USES
- Bladder outlet obstruction from benign prostatic hyperplasia
- Male pattern baldness

ADRs
- Decreased libido
- Impotence

α₁-Adrenergic Receptor Antagonists

DOXAZOSIN, PRAZOSIN, TAMSULOSIN

MOA
- Decreases smooth muscle tone in prostate and bladder (effect requires weeks)

USES
- Bladder outlet obstruction from increased urethral resistance such as benign prostatic hyperplasia

ADRs
- Orthostatic hypotension and syncope
- Blurred vision
- Headache

Renin-Angiotensin-Aldosterone System

The renin-angiotensin-aldosterone system (RAAS) plays a fundamental role in the physiological regulation of blood pressure (BP). The RAAS pathway is activated in response to decreased blood pressure.

Activation of the RAAS pathway

1. Decreased BP is sensed by the kidney and the carotid sinus
1a. Decreased BP and the kidney
- In the kidney, decreased BP is sensed by the macula densa cells located in the proximal segment of the distal convoluted tubule
- Cyclooxygenase (COX) enzyme is activated and results in production of prostaglandins and subsequent stimulation for the release of the peptide, renin, from juxtaglomerular (JG) cells located in the arterioles of the nephron

1b. Decreased BP and the carotid sinus
- The carotid sinus also detects decreased BP and results in activation of the sympathetic nervous system. Activation of the sympathetic nervous system results in the activation of β_1-adrenoreceptors in the heart and kidney. Activation of β_1-adrenoreceptors in the heart results in increased cardiac output and increased BP. Activation of β_1-adrenoreceptors in the kidney results in the release of renin from JG cells

2. Conversion of angiotensin I to angiotensin II
- Renin released by the JG cells facilitates the conversion of the inactive plasma protein, angiotensinogen (produced in the liver) to angiotensin I (AGI)
- AGI is converted to angiotensin II (AGII) by the enzyme, angiotensin converting enzyme (ACE)

3. Regulation of BP by AGII
3a. Stimulation of aldosterone secretion
- AGII stimulates the synthesis and release of the hormone, aldosterone from the adrenal gland
- Aldosterone secretion results in increased renal tubular Na^+ reabsorption and increased renal tubular secretion of K^+ and H^+
- Increased Na^+ and water retention results in increased BP

3b. Stimulation of vasopressin secretion
- AGII binds to and subsequently activates angiotensin receptors in the hypothalamus and posterior pituitary
- Activation of angiotensin receptors results in the synthesis and release of vasopressin, also known as antidiuretic hormone (ADH)
- ADH stimulates renal tubular water reabsorption which results in increased BP

3c. Induction of vasoconstriction
- AGII is one of the most potent endogenous vasoconstrictors in humans
- Increased vasoconstriction results in increased BP

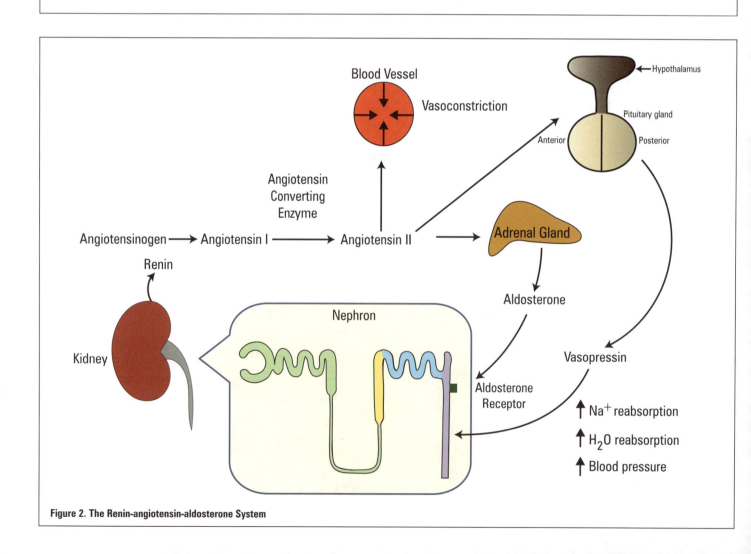

Figure 2. The Renin-angiotensin-aldosterone System

Renin-Angiotensin-Aldosterone System

ACE Inhibitors

CAPTOPRIL, LISINOPRIL

MOA
- Prevents conversion AGI → AGII by inhibiting angiotensin converting enzyme (ACE)

USES
- Congestive heart failure
- Hypertension
- CAPTOPRIL – LV cardiac dysfunction
- CAPTOPRIL – Diabetic nephropathy
- LISINOPRIL – Acute MI

PK CAPTOPRIL
- Short $t_{1/2}$ (less than 3 hours)

PK LISINOPRIL
- Long $t_{1/2}$ (12 hours)

ADRs
- Angioedema
- Cough
- Hyperkalemia
- Hypotension
- Altered sense of taste
- Gynecomastia
- Proteinuria
- Nausea
- Dizziness
- Headache
- Vomiting

CONTRAINDICATIONS
- Pregnancy-oligohydramnios
- Renal insufficiency

Vasopressin Receptor Agonist

DESMOPRESSIN

MOA
- A synthetic analogue of the natural human hormone, 8-arginine vasopressin, also known as ADH
- Vasopressin type 2 (V2) receptor agonist
- Increases water reabsorption in the renal tubule

USES
- Hemophilia A, with factor VII levels greater than 5%
- Neurohypophyseal diabetes insipidus
- Primary nocturnal enuresis
- von Willebrand disease type 1 (mild to moderate), with factor VIII levels greater than 5%

PK
- Short $t_{1/2}$ (1-2.5 hours)

ADRs
- Fatigue
- Flushing
- Hyponatremia
- Muscle cramps
- Nausea
- Palpitations
- Tachyarrhythmia
- Vomiting
- Water intoxication

Vasopressin Receptor Antagonists

TOLVAPTAN

MOA
- Vasopressin type 2 (V2) receptor antagonist
- Vasopressin antagonism → increased renal excretion of water → decreased urine osmolality, increased serum sodium concentration

USES
- Euvolemia
- Hyponatremia
- Hypervolemia

PK
- Long $t_{1/2}$ (12 hours)

ADRs
- Asthenia
- Constipation
- Dizziness
- Hyperglycemia
- Hypovolemia
- Nausea
- Polyuria
- Thirst
- Xerostomia

NSAIDs
- See Central Nervous System Chapter
- Inhibits prostaglandin synthesis → decreased release of renin

Angiotensin Receptor Antagonist

LOSARTAN

MOA
- Angiotensin type 1 (AT1) receptor antagonist
- Angiotensin II antagonism → decreased vasoconstriction and aldosterone secretion

USES
- Cerebrovascular accident (LVH)
- Diabetic nephropathy
- Hypertension

PK
- Short $t_{1/2}$ (2 hours)

ADRs
- Asthenia
- Diarrhea
- Dizziness
- Hypotension
- Angioedema
- Cough

CONTRAINDICATIONS
- Pregnancy-oligohydramnios
- Renal insufficiency

Renin Inhibitors

ALISKIREN

MOA
- Direct inhibitor of renin

USES
- Hypertension

PK
- Long $t_{1/2}$ (40 hours)

ADRs
- Angioedema of face, lips, tongue, glottis and/or larynx, extremities
- Diarrhea
- Persistent cough
- Rash

CONTRAINDICATIONS
- Pregnancy-oligohydramnios

β-Blockers
- See Cardiovascular Drugs chapter
- Inhibits $β_1$-adrenoreceptors located on JG cells → inhibits release of renin

Diuretics

Key Principles in the Pharmacology of Diuretics

- Diuretics are agents that facilitate the rate of urine output by affecting solute reabsorption
- Diuretics allow for the elimination of excess water from the body in conditions such as congestive heart failure and hypertension
- There are 2 main mechanisms of action of diuretics: (1) inhibition of renal tubular reabsorption of Na^+ and (2) production of hyperosmolic environment in the renal tubule
- The inhibition of Na^+ reabsorption at specific sites along the nephron is the most common mechanism of action of diuretics

EFFECTS OF THE INHIBITION OF NA+ REABSORPTION IN THE NEPHRON

1. The inhibition of Na^+ at proximal segments of the nephron will promote Na^+ reabsorption at distal segments of the nephron, especially the cortical collecting duct
    - Carbonic anhydrase inhibitors (CAIs) inhibit Na^+ reabsorption at the proximal convoluted tubule (PCT) which results in the reabsorption of Na^+ at distal segments of the nephron. Therefore, while CAIs are potent inhibitors of Na^+ reabsorption, they have reduced efficacy as diuretics
    - Diuretics that induce reabsorption of Na^+ from sections of the nephron that are proximal to the cortical collecting duct (CCD) will result in increased reabsorption of Na^+ at the CCD. Such diuretics produce a predictable ADR profile of potassium-wasting (discussed below) and are consequently labelled, potassium-wasting diuretics

2. The inhibition of Na^+ reabsorption can also disrupt the handling of other electrolytes

HCO_3^- AND Cl^-

- The inhibition of HCO_3^- reabsorption in the nephron results in the decreased secretion and subsequent accumulation of Cl^- in the body resulting in a **hyperchloremic** state, while reabsorption of HCO_3^- in the nephron results in increased Cl^- secretion resulting in a **hypochloremic** state
- The inhibition or induction of HCO_3^- secretion in the nephron affects the Cl^- concentration in the body because of the HCO_3^-/Cl^- anion exchanger located in the basolateral surface of cells of the PCT and CCD. The HCO_3^-/Cl^- anion exchanger exchanges HCO_3^- for Cl^- during HCO_3^- reabsorption

POTASSIUM-WASTING AND SPARING DIURETICS

- Diuretics that promote Na^+ reabsorption at segments of the nephron that are proximal to the CCD result in increased loss of K^+ in the urine and a **hypokalemic** state. Such diuretics are referred to as **potassium-wasting diuretics**
- In contrast to the above, diuretics that promote Na^+ reabsorption at the CCD result in decreased loss of K^+ in the urine and a **hyperkalemic** state. Such diuretics are referred to a **potassium-sparing diuretics**

THE EPITHELIAL NA+ CHANNEL (ENaC)

- ENaC is located in the apical membrane of the principle cells of the CCD
- ENaC transports Na^+ into the renal tubule
- The transport of Na^+ by ENaC results in an excess of negatively charged ions in the urine and a net negative charge in the urine → increased secretion of positively charged K^+ and H^+ into the urine → secretion of H^+ into the urine results in the reabsorption of HCO_3^- from the urine → reabsorption of HCO_3^- from the urine results in the secretion of Cl^- into the urine through the action of the HCO_3^-/Cl^- anion exchanger. The result is **hypokalemic hypochloremic metabolic alkalosis**
- Potassium-wasting diuretics that inhibit Na^+ at segments of the nephron that are proximal to the CCD will result in increased Na^+ transport by ENaC located in the cells of the CCD and induction of **hypokalemic hypochloremic metabolic alkalosis**
- Conversely, potassium-sparing diuretics that act directly on the cells of CCD and block Na^+ reabsorption through inhibition of ENaC will produce an effect opposite to that described above for transport of Na^+ by ENaC and will result in **hyperkalemic hyperchloremic metabolic acidosis**
- CAIs are potassium-wasting diuretics; however, they do not tend to induce the typical **hypokalemic hypochloremic metabolic alkalosis** induced by other potassium-wasting diuretics because CAIs are potent inhibitors of HCO_3^- reabsorption at the PCT. Decreased reabsorption of HCO_3^- at the PCT results in decreased secretion of Cl^- into the urine. The decreased reabsorption of HCO_3^- and decreased secretion of Cl^- at the PCT results in an excess of HCO_3^- in the urine and an excess of Cl^- in serum that cannot be corrected through the exchange of HCO_3^- and Cl^- by the HCO_3^-/Cl^- anion exchanger at the CCD. The net result is **hypokalemic hyperchloremic metabolic acidosis**

All diuretics can cause electrolyte abnormalities and hypovolemia, which in turn leads to orthostasis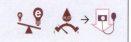

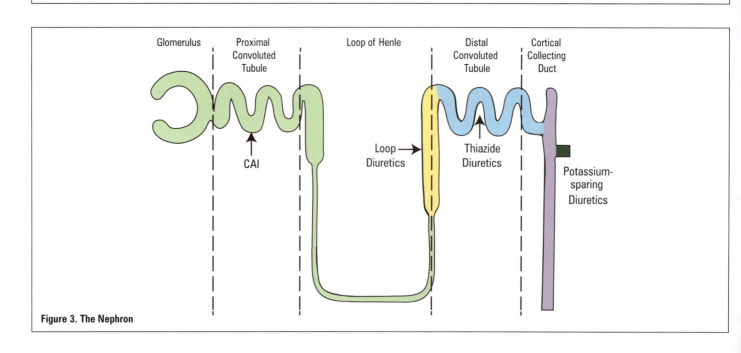

Figure 3. The Nephron

Carbonic Anhydrase Inhibitors (CAIs)
(Potassium-Wasting Diuretics)

CAIs induce diuresis by inhibiting the enzyme, carbonic anhydrase (CA). The precise mechanism of action of CAIs is complex, but can be better understood by knowing the following:
1. HCO_3^- can only be transported into cells after it is converted to gaseous CO_2. Gaseous CO_2 diffuses into the cell
2. CA catalyzes the conversion of HCO_3^- to H_2O and CO_2
3. Once diffused into the cell, CO_2 is converted to $H_2CO_3^-$ and H^+ through the action of CA, leading to the production of HCO_3^- and H^+
4. Intracellular HCO_3^- is reabsorbed into the serum and H^+ is secreted into the urine by the Na^+/H^+ antiporter in exchange for Na^+
5. Inhibition of CA by CAIs result in decreased availability of H^+ and decreased exchange of H^+ and Na^+ by the Na^+/H^+ antiporter. The result is decreased Na^+ reabsorption. The inhibition of CA by CAIs also result in decreased HCO_3^- reabsorption

With the introduction of safer and more efficaceous diuretics, the most common use of CAIs is as now a topical agent for the treatment of glaucoma. The cells of the ciliary body secrete aqueous humor into the eye by a mechanism that is dependent on the enzymatic activity of CA. In glaucoma, the production of aqueous humor in the eye can be reduced by inhibiting CA activity with CAIs.

ACETAZOLAMIDE
MOA
- Inhibition of CA → decreased production of H^+ and HCO_3^- → decreased H^+ secretion, increased Na^+, K^+, HCO_3^- and water excretion at the renal proximal tubules → alkaline diuresis

USES
- Acute mountain sickness (HACE, HAPE)
- Edema
- Epilepsy
- **Glaucoma**
- Urine alkalinization

PK
- Moderate $t_{1/2}$ (4-6 hours)

ADRs
- **Hypokalemic hyperchloremic metabolic acidosis**
- Alteration of taste sense
- Confusion
- Diarrhea
- Anorexia
- Nausea
- Sulfonamide adverse reaction (e.g. Stevens-Johnson syndrome, toxic epidermal necrolysis, hepatic necrosis)
- Tinnitus
- Weight loss

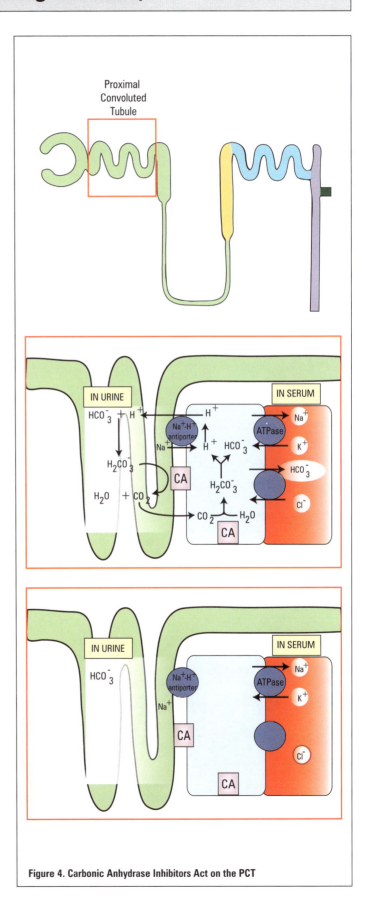

Figure 4. Carbonic Anhydrase Inhibitors Act on the PCT

Loop Diuretics

Loop diuretics induce diuresis by inhibiting the Na+/K+/2Cl− symporter in the thick ascending limb (TAL) of the Loop of Henle. Loop diuretics cause the greatest excretion of salt and water (i.e. are the most potent) because of the relatively high Na+ concentration in this segment.

The transport of Na+, K+ and 2Cl− by the Na+/K+/2Cl− symporter usually results in a neutral charge in the urine because 2 positive (Na+ and K+) and 2 negative (2Cl−) charged ions are removed from the urine. However, the transport of Na+, K+ and 2Cl− by the Na+/K+/2Cl− symporter results in the transport of a positively charged K+ back into the urine and results in a net positive charge in the urine. The positive charge in the urine drives the reabsorption of positively charged Ca^{2+} and Mg^{2+} via paracellular transport. The inhibition of the Na+/K+/2Cl− symporter by loop diuretics results in decreased absorption of Na+ and other ions including K+, Cl−, Ca^{2+} and Mg^{2+}.

The TAL of the loop of Henle is located within the medulla of the kidney. Na+ reabsorption by the Na+/K+/2Cl− symporter contributes to the establishment of the medullary concentration gradient and the production of concentrated urine in the collecting duct. The inhibition of the Na+/K+/2Cl− symporter by loop diuretics results in depletion of the medullary concentration gradient and less ADH-induced water reabsorption in the collecting tubule.

Loop diuretics may induce ototoxicity because maintenance of the endolymph ionic concentration is dependent on a functioning Na+/K+/2Cl− symporter. The inhibition of the Na+/K+/2Cl− symporter with loop diuretic disturbs the endolymph ionic concentration and results in sensorineural hearing loss that is typically reversible.

FUROSEMIDE

MOA
- Inhibits the Na+/K+/2Cl− symporter to reduce salt reabsorption which draws water into the lumen

USES
- Edema
- Hypertension
- Pulmonary edema
- Acute hypercalcemia

PK
- Short $t_{1/2}$ (2 hours)

ADRs
- Headache
- Hyperchloremic metabolic alkalosis
- Hyperglycemia
- Hyperuricemia
- Gout
- Ototoxicity
- Bladder spasms
- Hypomagnesemia
- Anorexia
- Paresthesia
- Scaling eczema

NOTES
- Other examples include **ETHACRYNIC ACID** and **TORSEMIDE**

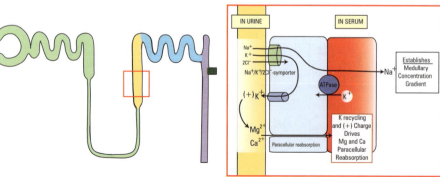
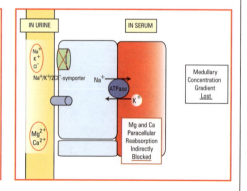

Figure 5. Loop Diuretics Act on the Thick Ascending Limb of the Loop of Henle

Thiazide Diuretics (Potassium-Wasting Diuretics)

Thiazide diuretics induce diuresis by inhibiting the Na^+/Cl^- symporter in the distal convoluted tubule (DCT). Compared to loop diuretics, thiazides are less effective since most Na^+ has already been absorbed proximal to the DCT. Thiazides also lead to increased Ca^{2+} reabsorption by the following:
1. The Na^+/Ca^{2+} antiporter located at the basolateral surface of the cell transports Na^+ out of the cells in exchange for Ca^{2+}
2. In the presence of thiazide diuretics, inhibition of Na^+ transport by the Na^+/Cl^- symporter results in a decrease in intracellular Na^+ as Na^+/K^+-ATPase continues to pump Na^+ out of the cell
3. Decreased intracellular Na^+ is replenished through the reversal of the Na^+/Ca^{2+} antiporter resulting in increased intracellular Na^+ and decreased intracellular Ca^{2+}
4. The decreased intracellular Ca^{2+} results in increased reabsorption of Ca^{2+} from the urine through the epithelial Ca^{2+} channel (ECaC)

HYDROCHLOROTHIAZIDE
MOA
- Inhibits Na^+/Cl^- symporter in the DCT → decreased renal tubular reabsorption of Na^+ and Cl^-, increased urinary excretion of Na^+ and water

USES
- Edema
- Hypertension
- Congestive heart failure

PK
- Long $t_{1/2}$ (5.6-14.8 h)

ADRs
- Gout
- Diarrhea
- Hyperchloremic metabolic alkalosis
- Hyperglycemia
- Hypotension
- Anorexia
- Photosensitivity
- Spasticity
- Vomiting
- Hypomagnesemia

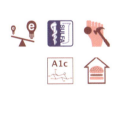

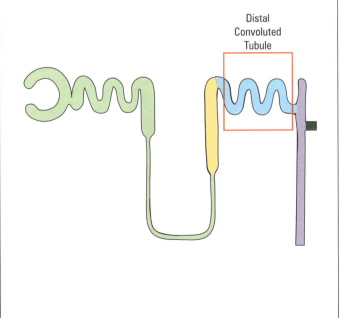

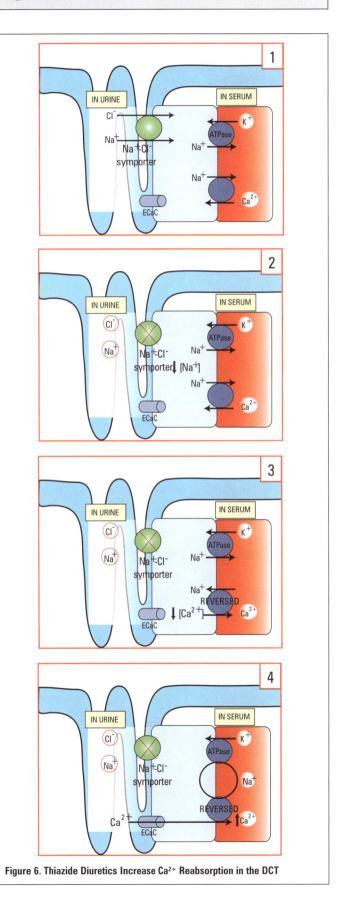

Figure 6. Thiazide Diuretics Increase Ca^{2+} Reabsorption in the DCT

Potassium-Sparing Diuretics

The potassium-sparing diuretics have previously been introduced as diuretics that inhibit Na^+ reabsorption by inhibiting the ENaC of the CCD and result in hyperkalemic hyperchloremic metabolic acidosis. The potassium-sparing diuretics either inhibit ENaC directly (e.g. **AMILORIDE, TRIAMTERENE**) or indirectly by down-regulating its synthesis through inhibition of the aldosterone receptor (e.g. **SPIRONOLACTONE**).

Caution must be exercised when potassium-sparing drugs are concurrently used with medications that inhibit aldosterone synthesis, namely ACE inhibitors, angiotensin receptor antagonists and β-blockers, as these agents also induce increased serum potassium.

AMILORIDE, TRIAMTERENE
MOA
- Inhibits the reabsorption of Na^+ in exchange for K^+ and H^+ in the renal tubule

USES
- Congestive heart failure
- Hypertension
- Edema

PK
- Moderate $t_{1/2}$ (6-9 hours)

ADRs
- **HYPERKALEMIA**
- Diarrhea
- Headache
- Anorexia
- Orthostatic hypotension
- Gout
- Photosensitivity (**TRIAMTERENE**)

SPIRONOLACTONE
MOA
- Aldosterone receptor antagonist that causes a decrease in the number of ENaC sodium potassium exchanges sites in the DCT → increased excretion of Na^+ and water, decreased excretion of K^+

USES
- Edema and/or ascites
- Hypertension
- Hypokalemia
- Primary aldosteronism

PK
- Short $t_{1/2}$ (1.4 hours)

ADRs
- **HYPERKALEMIA**
- Abnormal menstruation
- Confusion
- Diarrhea
- Dizziness
- Gynecomastia
- Headache
- Lethargy

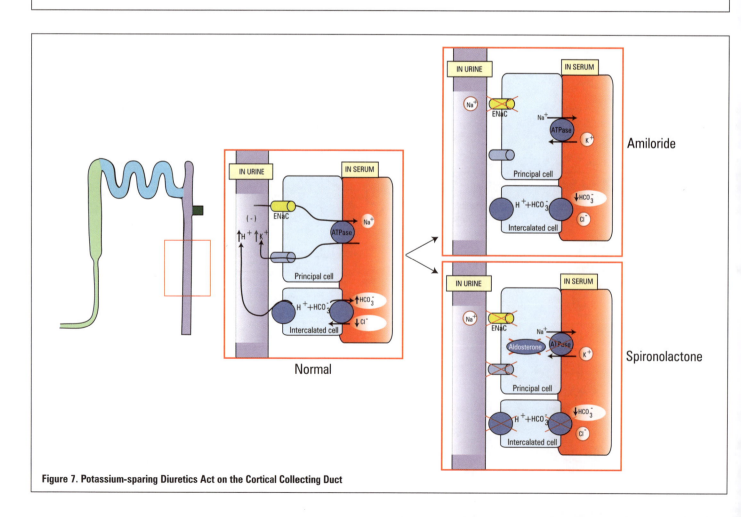

Figure 7. Potassium-sparing Diuretics Act on the Cortical Collecting Duct

Osmotic Diuretics

Osmotic diuretics are osmotic agents that are freely filtered by the glomerulus and result in hyperosmolality of the glomerular filtrate which results in decreased water reabsorption along the nephron. Osmotic diuretics also work systemically before arriving at the kidney. Osmotic diuretics increase the intravascular volume by extracting water from various body fluid compartments. The expansion of the intravascular volume is a greater therapeutic benefit compared to the diuretic effect of these agents. For example, the extraction of intracellular water by agents such as osmotic diuretics aid in the alleviation of increased pressure in the respective fluid compartments that exists in pathological conditions such as glaucoma and elevated intracranial pressure. Additionally, osmotic diuretics can be effective for the extraction of water into the intravascular space in some forms of shock, where fluids are mal-distributed from the plasma into the interstitium. The extraction of water into the intravascular space helps to maintain the effective arterial volume in such conditions. Systemically, the expansion of intravascular volume induced by osmotic diuretics can cause hyponatremia due to the dilution of plasma Na^+. Conversely, in the nephron, their diuretic effect can cause dehydration and hypernatremia due to the concentration of plasma Na^+.

In contrast to the majority of diuretics, osmotic diuretics are contraindicated in congestive heart failure because they can exacerbate fluid overloaded states through the expansion of intravascular volume.

MANNITOL

MOA
- **MANNITOL** is freely filtered by the glomerulus and not reabsorbed along the nephron which results in hyperosmolality of the glomerular filtrate → increased water excretion, decreased renal tubular absorption of Na^+, Cl^- and other solutes

USES
- Acute renal failure
- Excretion of toxic drugs that are eliminated in the urine
- Increased intracranial pressure
- Increased intraocular pressure
- Irrigation of urinary bladder
- Measurement of renal clearance

PK
- Moderate $t_{1/2}$ (4.7 hours)

ADRs
- Chest pain
- Headache
- Hypotension
- Nausea
- Urinary retention
- Vomiting

Erectile Dysfunction

Erection Physiology

- Sexual stimulation induces the release of nitric oxide (NO)
- NO activates guanylyl cyclase
- Guanylyl cyclase catalyzes the formation of the intracellular second messenger, cyclic guanosine monophosphate (cGMP)
- cGMP decreases intracellular calcium
- Decreased intracellular calcium levels results in smooth muscle relaxation and increased blood flow to the penis resulting in erection

Phosphodiesterase Type-5 (PDE5) Inhibitors

SILDENAFIL, TADALAFIL, VARDENAFIL

MOA
- Inhibiton of PDE5 → increase in intracellular cGMP → smooth muscle relaxation and vasodilation

USES
- Erectile dysfunction
- Pulmonary hypertension

PK SILDENAFIL
- Moderate $t_{1/2}$ (3-5 hours)

PK TADALAFIL
- Long $t_{1/2}$ (17.5 hours)

PK VARDENAFIL
- Moderate $t_{1/2}$ (4-5 hours)

ADRs
- Flushing
- Headache
- Dyspnea
- Epistaxis
- Erythema
- Insomnia
- Dyspepsia
- Rhinitis
- Dizziness
- Tinnitus

CONTRAINDICATIONS
- Nitrate therapy for angina pectoris or selective α_1 adrenergic blockers for hypertension (concurrent use of these therapeutics results in hypotension and shock)

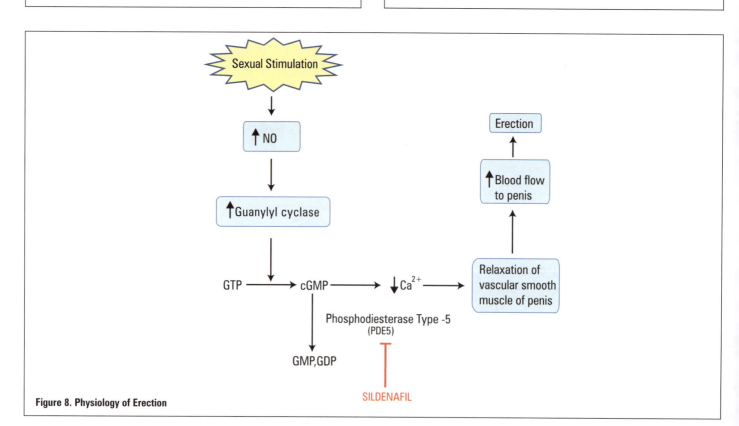

Figure 8. Physiology of Erection

Respiratory Drugs

Chapter Authors: Andrew W. Browne, Moumita Sarkar and David Simpson

Faculty Reviewers: Andrea Gershon and Geert W. 't Jong

IN THIS CHAPTER

Asthma 154
    Short Term Relievers
    Long Term Controllers

Antihistamines 157

DRUGS IN THIS CHAPTER

Generic Name	US Trade Name	Canadian Trade Name
albuterol (salbutamol)	ACCUNEB, PROVENTIL, VENTOLIN, VOSPIRE, PROAIR	AIROMIR, COMBIVENT, VENTOLIN
aminophylline	NORPHYL, PHYLLOCONTIN, TRUPHYLLINE	PHYLLOCONTIN
beclomethasone	BECLOVENT, BECONASE, QVAR, VANCENASE	PROPADERM, QVAR, RIVANASE
cetirizine	ZYRTECT	REACTINE, ZYRTECT
chlorpheniramine	ALLER-CHLOR, CPM, CHLORPHEN, TELDRIN	BENYLIN, DRISTAN, CORICIDIN, ROBITUSSIN, SINUTAB, TRIAMINIC
cromolyn	CROLOM, GASTROCROM, INTAL, NASALCROM	CROMOLYN, NALCROM, OPTICROM, RHINARIS
desloratadine	CLARINEX	AERIUS
dimenhydrinate	DRAMAMINE, DRIMINATE, HYDRATE, MOTION SICKNESS, TRIPTONE	GRAVOL
diphenhydramine	BENADRYL, BENYLIN, DIPHENHIST, DIPHENYL, GENAHIST, GERIDRYL, NYTOL	ALLERGY, ALLERNIX, ALMINIL, BENADRYL, BENYLIN, BUCKLEY'S BEDTIME, ERGODRYL, SIMPLY SLEEP, SINUTAB, SLEEP AID, UNISOM
fexofenadine	ALLEGRA	
fluticasone	VERAMYST, CUTIVATE, FLONASE, FLOVENT, ADVAIR	AVAMYS, ADVAIR, FLONASE, FLOVENT
formoterol	FORADIL, PERFOROMIST	FORADIL, OXEZE, SYMBICORT
ipratropium	ATROVENT, COMBIVENT, DUONEB	COMBIVENT, DUOVENT
loratadine	ALAVERT, CLARITIN, CLEARATADINE	CLARITIN
montelukast	SINGULAIR	
nedocromil	ALOCRIL	
prednisone	DELTASONE, PREDNICOT, STERAPRED	WINPRED
promethazine	ANTINAUS, PHENADOZ, PHENERGAN, PROMACOT, PROMETHEGAN, PROREX	PHENERGAN, PROMATUSSIN
salmeterol	ADVAIR, SEREVENT	
terbutaline	BRETHINE	BRICANYL
theophylline	THEO-24, UNIPHYL, THEO-DUR, THEO-TIME, THEOCAP, THEOCHRON, ELIXOPHYLLIN, QUIBRON-T	THEOLAIR, UNIPHYL
tiotropium	SPIRIVA	
zafirlukast	ACCOLATE	
zileuton	ZYFLO	

Asthma

- **Asthma** is characterized by reversible airflow obstruction, bronchial hyperresponsiveness, airway inflammation, mucus plugging and smooth muscle hypertrophy
- For many, asthma begins in infancy and early childhood through a complex interplay of genetic and environmental factors
- Asthmatic patients may suffer from unpredictable, disabling attacks characterized by severe dyspnea, coughing, wheezing and bronchospasms

Immunopathogenesis
- Exposure to allergen → IgE synthesis → IgE binds to mast cells in the airway mucosa
- Re-exposure to allergen → IgE-mediated release of chemical mediators from from T cells and mast cells:
    - Histamine, tryptase, prostaglandin D_2 (PGD2), leukotriene C_4, and platelet-activating factor (PAF)
- Mediators provoke contraction of airway smooth muscle, causing the immediate fall in the forced expiratory volume in one second (FEV_1)
- Cytokines attract and activate eosinophils and neutrophils
- Cellular infiltration contributes to the edema, mucus hypersecretion, smooth muscle contraction, and increase in bronchial reactivity associated with the late asthmatic response, and results in a second fall in FEV_1 hours after exposure
- In addition to direct antigenic-mediated release, inhaled irritants can stimulate neuronal pathways to trigger indirect mediator release from mast cells to provoke bronchoconstriction

Asthma exacerbation can be divided into:
- Two phases
    1. Early response – within minutes
    2. Late response – hours after exposure
- Two components
    1. Obstruction – reversible bronchial smooth muscle contraction and airway hyperreactivity
    2. Inflammation – mucosal thickening and airway secretions
- Two broad etiologies
    1. Intrinsic – non-immune mediated (irritant provoked)
    2. Extrinsic – immune mediated response (allergic, IgE)
        - Extrinsic factors produce an intrinsic immune response

Treatment
- Short-term relievers
    - Immediate reversal of smooth muscle contraction
- Long-term controllers
    - Sustained reversal of inflammation, edema and cellular infiltration

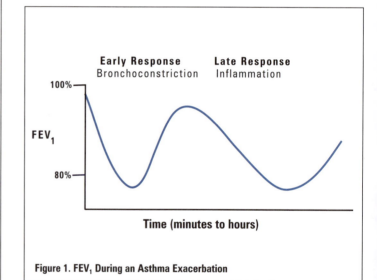

Figure 1. FEV_1 During an Asthma Exacerbation

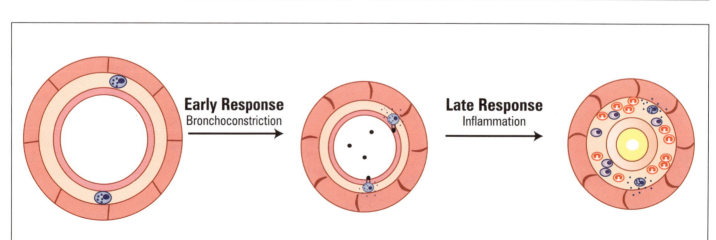

Figure 2. Airway Pathophysiology in an Asthma Exacerbation

Asthma Short Term Relievers

These medications may be used to manage the emergent symptoms of asthma

CLASS Ia

Short-acting β₂-agonists

ALBUTEROL, TERBUTALINE

MOA
- Stimulates β₂-receptors → activates GTP-binding proteins → increases adenylate cyclase activity → increases cAMP levels → relaxation of bronchial smooth muscle

USES
- DOC for acute exacerbations of intermittent asthma episodes
- Exercise and allergen-induced asthma (prophylaxis)
- COPD

PK ALBUTEROL
- Moderate $t_{1/2}$ (4-6 hours)
- Can be administered by inhalation, IV, or orally

PK TERBUTALINE
- Oral administration – short $t_{1/2}$ (3-4 hours)
- Subcutaneous administration – moderate/long $t_{1/2}$ (3-14 hours)

CLASS Ib

Long-acting β₂-agonists

SALMETEROL, FORMOTEROL

MOA
- Same as above

USES
- Maintenance therapy for asthma
- COPD
- Exercise-induced asthma

PK SALMETEROL
- Moderate $t_{1/2}$ (5-6 hours)
- Slow onset, not useful for acute asthmatic attacks

PK FORMOTEROL
- Moderate $t_{1/2}$ (10 hours)
- More rapid onset than **SALMETEROL**

ADRs
- Cardiac stimulation (cross-reactivity for β₁-receptors)
- Tachycardia, palpitations, arrhythmias
- Muscle tremor
- Mild to moderate hyperglycemia and hypokalemia (systemic effects)

CLASS II

Anticholinergics

IPRATROPIUM

MOA
- Competitive muscarinic receptor antagonist
- Blocks vagal-mediated bronchoconstriction and mucus secretion

USES
- First line use for COPD
- Exacerbation of asthma
- Enhances effects of β₂-agonists in acute severe asthma

PK
- Short $t_{1/2}$ (2-4 hours)

ADRs
- Anti-BLUSHPADS BBC (please see Autonomic Drugs chapter)

NOTES
- **TIOTROPIUM** is in the same class but is only indicated for second line use for moderate COPD

CLASS III

Methylxanthines

THEOPHYLLINE, AMINOPHYLLINE

MOA
- Unclear – adenosine receptor or PDE inhibition → increases cAMP levels
- Causes bronchodilation and can increase the force of contraction of the diaphragmatic muscles

USES
- 2nd or 3rd line agent for asthma, COPD

PK
- Variable elimination $t_{1/2}$ – dependent on type of population and indication

ADRs: VERY Narrow Therapeutic Index
- CNS stimulation → headaches, nervousness, seizures, insomnia
- Cardiac stimulation → palpitations, arrhythmias, PVCs
- GI irritation → abdominal pain, increases acid secretion, anorexia

NOTES
- Should monitor serum **THEOPHYLLINE** levels
- Several known drug interactions
- **AMINOPHYLLINE** is composed of **THEOPHYLLINE** and diethylamine

Asthma Long Term Controllers

These medications are used to prevent asthma attacks

CLASS IV

Corticosteroids

BECLOMETHASONE, FLUTICASONE, PREDNISONE

MOA
- Reduces inflammation and hyperreactivity, and promotes epithelial regeneration

USES
- DOC for chronic asthma therapy
- Very effective in improving all indices of asthma control
- Rhinitis (allergic or non-allergic)
- Treatment of COPD in certain patients

PK BECLOMETHASONE
- Short $t_{1/2}$ (3 hours)
- Given by inhalation

PK FLUTICASONE PROPIONATE
- Moderate $t_{1/2}$ (7-8 hours for both inhaled and intravenous administration)

PK PREDNISONE
- Short $t_{1/2}$ (1 hour)
- Given orally or by IV

ADRs: MANY with oral or IV administration
(see Immune Response Modifiers chapter)
- <u>Oral candidiasis (thrush), hoarseness</u>
- Adrenal suppression – weakness, fatigue, and muscle loss
- Slowed growth rate in children
- Cataracts, glaucoma
- Skin thinning, bruising
- Osteoporosis
- Immunosuppression

NOTES
- Less ADRs are assocated with inhaled corticosteroids compared to the oral route

CLASS V

Leukotriene Pathway Inhibitors

MONTELUKAST, ZAFIRLUKAST, ZILEUTON
- Leukotriene pathway inhibitors reduce leukotriene-induced bronchoconstriction, airway hyperreactivity and edema

MOA
MONTELUKAST, ZAFIRLUKAST
- Inhibition of leukotriene D_4 receptor binding preventing airway edema, smooth muscle contraction and other respiratory inflammation

ZILEUTON
- Inhibition of 5-lipoxygenase – prevents leukotriene synthesis

USES
- Asthma
- Can be added to treatment with inhaled steroids
- Especially effective for aspirin-induced asthma

PK MONTELUKAST
- Short/moderate $t_{1/2}$ (3-5 hours)

PK ZAFIRLUKAST
- Moderate $t_{1/2}$ (10 hours)

CLASS VI

Cromolyns

CROMOLYN, NEDOCROMIL

MOA
- Alters function of delayed chloride channels and inhibits activation of mast cells

USES
- Asthma
- Exercise induced asthma
- Nasal spray/eye drops for allergic rhinitis and conjunctivitis

Antihistamines

Histamine

- Synthesized from the amino acid histidine
- Stored in granules, primarily in mast cells and basophils
- Rapidly inactivated by enzymatic metabolism

- Concentrated in:
  1. Tissues with large mast cell numbers → lung, skin, nose, GI, mouth, feet and blood vessels (anything that touches the outside world and blood – sites of potential injury)
  2. Enterochromaffin-like (ECL) cells – stomach fundus

- Bound to sulfated polysaccharides in granules that also contain ATP and other mediators (autocoids)
- Increased secretion occurs in certain neoplasms with increased mast cell or basophil number (e.g. gastric carcinoid, systemic mastocytosis)

Histamine Release
1. Immunological release
   - Antigen-IgE immunoglobulin complex mediated degranulation (exocytotic)
   - Process requires energy and calcium
   - Degranulation is inhibited by:
     - Asthma drugs
       - CROMOLYN, THEOPHYLLINE, β_2-agonists
     - Histamine binding to H_2-receptors on mast cells
       - Negative feedback control
2. Chemical and mechanical release
   - Direct release or displacement of histamine from cells (non-exocytotic) – cannot be inhibited
   - Drug-induced displacement does NOT require energy nor degranulation
     - MORPHINE, TUBOCURARINE, SUCCINYLCHOLINE
   - Additional causes of degranulation
     - Mechanical/thermal stress
     - Radiation
     - Venoms (bees and snakes)
     - Cytotoxic compounds (idiosyncratic)
     - X-ray contrast media (idiosyncratic)

NOTES
- H_2-receptor antagonists can be found in the Gastrointestinal Drugs chapter

H_1-receptor Mechanism of Action
- H_1-receptors associate with intracellular G proteins
- $G\alpha_q$ activates phospholipase C which produces IP_3 and DAG
- Intracellular calcium increases

H_1-receptor Locations (Ubiquitous)
- Bronchial smooth muscle – constriction (particularly in asthma)
- Postsynaptic sensory nerve terminals – itching and pain
- Blood vessels – endothelial cell contraction and vasodilation (flushing, headache, shock, edema)
- Pregnant uterus – smooth muscle contraction (abortion)
- Intestinal smooth muscle – contractions (increased motility, diarrhea)
- Exocrine glands – increased secretion (nose, eyes, lungs, etc.)
- Cardiac atrial muscle – heart block or arrhythmias
- Brain neurotransmitter – post-synaptic membranes

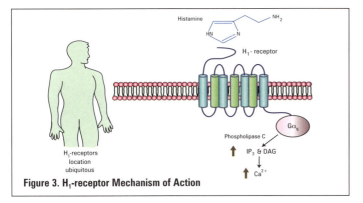

Figure 3. H_1-receptor Mechanism of Action

CLASS VIIIa

H_1-receptor Antagonist (1st Generation)

DIPHENHYDRAMINE, CHLORPHENIRAMINE, DIMENHYDRINATE, PROMETHAZINE

- Oral antihistamines, particularly H_1-receptor antagonists, have some anti-cholinergic activity and are sedating, making them useful for the control of pruritus

MOA
- Reversible-competitive antagonists of H_1-receptors
- Penetrate CNS well

USES
- Direct Effects (DIPHENHYDRAMINE, CHLORPHENIRAMINE)
  - Allergies → rhinitis and conjunctivitis, urticaria (hives), pruritus
- Indirect Effects
  - Insomnia – sedation via muscarinic receptors
  - Motion sickness, vertigo, nausea
  - Antiemetic
  - Pregnancy morning sickness
  - Treat Parkinson-like drug-induced extrapyramidal symptoms caused by antipsychotic drugs (anticholinergic effect)

PK
- Widely distributed – including CNS, placenta, breast milk

ADRs
- CNS sedation (additive with other sedatives)
- Paradoxical CNS stimulation (mainly in infants and young children)
- Fatigue, headache (vasodilation)
- Anticholinergic effects (atropine-like)

CLASS VIIIb

H_1-receptor Antagonists (2nd Generation-Non Sedating)

FEXOFENADINE, CETIRIZINE, LORATADINE, DESLORATADINE

MOA
- Reversible-competitive antagonists of H_1-receptors
- Penetrate CNS poorly → target peripheral over central H_1-receptors

USES
- Allergies → rhinitis, conjunctivitis, urticaria, pruritus
- Little value in asthma (symptom treatment only)

PK
- Poor CNS penetration
- FEXOFENADINE
  - Long $t_{1/2}$ (14 hours)
- CETIRIZINE
  - Moderate $t_{1/2}$ (8 hours)
- LORATADINE
  - Moderate $t_{1/2}$ (8 hours)
- DESLORATADINE
  - Long $t_{1/2}$ (28 hours)

ADRs
- Headaches

Appendix A

Tricks for Remembering Drug Names

Note: Drugs in the same therapeutic class often have similar endings, but there are exceptions.

Ending	Therapeutic Class	Examples
-afil	PDE-5 inhibitors	sildenafil, tadalafil, vardenafil
-ane	inhaled general anesthetics	halothane, enflurane, isoflurane
-artan	angiotensin receptor blockers	losartan, irbesartan, valsartan
-ase	thrombolytics	streptokinase, alteplase
-azole	antifungals	ketoconazole, itraconazole, fluconazole
-ceph/-cef	cephalosporin antibiotics	cephalexin, cefuroxime, ceftazidime
-cillin	penicillin antibiotics	penicillin, amoxicillin, cloxacillin
-cycline	tetracycline antibiotics	tetracycline, doxycycline, minocycline
-dipine	calcium channel blockers	nifedipine, felodipine, amlodipine
-dronate	bisphosphonates	alendronate, etidronate, risedronate
-floxacin	fluoroquinolone antibiotics	ciprofloxacin, norfloxacin, moxifloxacin
-lol	β-adrenergic antagonists	propranolol, metoprolol, labetalol
-micin/-mycin	aminoglycoside antibiotics	gentamicin, neomycin, tobramycin
-(par)in	anticoagulants	heparin, warfarin, enoxaprin
-prazole	proton pump inhibitors	omeprazole, pantoprazole, lansoprazole
-pril	ACE inhibitors	captopril, enalapril, lisinopril
-(s)one	corticosteroids	cortisone, prednisone, prednisolone
-statin	HMG-CoA reductase inhibitors	atorvastatin, lovastatin, pravastatin
-terol	bronchodilators	salmeterol, formoterol, albuterol
-thromycin	macrolide antibiotics	erythromycin, clarithromycin, azithromycin
-tidine	H_2-receptor antagonist	cimetidine, ranitidine, famotidine
-zepam/zolam	benzodiazepines	midazolam, diazepam, lorazepam
-zosin	α-adrenergic blockers	prazosin, terazosin, doxazosin